HEALTH AND LIFESTYLE WORKBOOK

HEALTH AND LIFESTYLE WORKBOOK

SECOND EDITION

Kathy McGinnis
San Diego City University

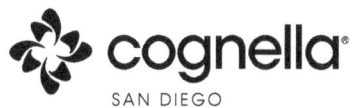

cognella®
SAN DIEGO

Bassim Hamadeh, CEO and Publisher
Mieka Portier, Senior Acquisitions Editor
Carrie Baarns, Manager, Revisions and Author Care
Kaela Martin, Project Editor
Alia Bales, Associate Production Manager
Emely Villavicencio, Senior Graphic Designer
Alexa Lucido, Licensing Manager
Natalie Piccotti, Director of Marketing
Kassie Graves, Senior Vice President of Editorial
Jamie Giganti, Director of Academic Publishing

cognella® | ACADEMIC PUBLISHING

3970 Sorrento Valley Blvd., Ste. 500, San Diego, CA 92121

CONTENTS

UNIT III.   Mental Health, Illness, and Addiction   29

UNIT IV. Complementary and Alternative Medicine, Aging, and Death 51

UNIT V. Human Sexuality 59

ACTIVE LEARNING

This book has interactive activities available to complement your reading.

Your instructor may have customized the selection of activities available for your unique course. Please check with your professor to verify whether your class will access this content through the Cognella

Active Learning portal (http://active.cognella.com) or through your home learning management system.

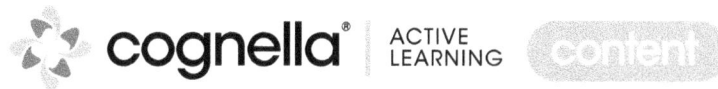

INTRODUCTION

H UMAN HEALTH IS A CONSTANTLY CHANGING subject. No single book could possibly cover every aspect of human health, but this workbook is meant to provide the student with an overview of the primary areas that affect our everyday lives. We learn via visual, auditory, and kinesthetic avenues, and this workbook is a kinesthetic tool, as writing down facts and concepts improves our ability to recall information. Using this workbook in unison with lecture materials provided by your instructor allows for an interactive experience throughout the semester. You will find that this is not your typical textbook, as it leaves space for note taking as more current information is added to the subject matter.

The subjects covered within the workbook include wellness, health care, mental health, complementary and alternative medicine, aging, death and dying, human sexuality, disease, and social violence. While there are many other topics that could be included here (environment, occupational hazards, and financial concerns), I have found these areas in particular to be more applicable to the average person—meaning that we experience issues within the areas covered, in some way, on a daily basis.

Along with this workbook is the Active Learning component supplied through the publisher. Access to active learning comes with the bundled package of book and access code. This site provides flashcards, subject-specific games, videos, quizzes, and assignments. All are designed to give the student another avenue for understanding the topics and preparing for exams.

Though we can't predict our future, we can take steps to improve our quality of life. I hope you find this book a helpful tool as you navigate the complexities of human health, both in the classroom and in your everyday life.

LANGUAGE OF HEALTH

CHAPTER 1

WELLNESS

HEALTH AND LIFESTYLES IS A COMPREHENSIVE course that covers the eight dimensions of wellness, focusing on an in-depth look at mental illness, aging, fitness and nutrition, complementary and alternative practices, communicable and noncommunicable diseases, drugs, alcohol, cannabis and tobacco, human sexuality, and social violence.

Health: A state of complete physical, mental, and social well-being and not merely the absence of disease

Wellness: Being in good health and an engaged member of a given society. Putting an emphasis on preventing illness and living a vital life

Dimensions of Wellness

There are eight dynamic and interrelated dimensions that are influenced by the personal decisions you make in your life. They are as follows:

Physical Wellness—maintaining a healthy body and seeking care when needed.

Emotional Wellness—understanding your feelings and coping effectively with stress.

Social Wellness—development of meaningful relationships with others and showing empathy.

Spiritual Wellness—constructing a set of values that help you seek meaning and purpose through relaxation and religion.

Intellectual Wellness—active participation in scholastic, cultural, and community activities. Always expanding on your knowledge base.

Environmental Wellness—encourages us to live in harmony with the Earth by taking actions to protect it.

Occupational Wellness—personal satisfaction and enhancement in one's life through work.

Financial Wellness—learning how to successfully manage finances (Life of Wellness Institute, 2021).

When evaluating these components in your life, do you see balance among all eight?

Homeostasis: From the Greek for "same" and "steady," meaning a balanced state.

Gratitude: An emotion with many benefits for those who practice it. Practicing gratitude improves our mental health and boosts our relationships with others. Scientific studies have shown that this powerful emotion can improve sleep, enhance romantic relationships, protect from illness, motivate us to exercise, and boost happiness.

Mindfulness: A person's active state of thoughtful existence. Someone practicing mindfulness is paying attention to the present, using all of their senses, and is aware of his or her thoughts and feelings without judgment.

Curiosity: Research suggests that curiosity keeps us sharp. It is a basic component of human nature. We have a natural desire for information. This mental trait motivates us. Benjamin Hayden, an assistant professor of brain and cognitive sciences at the University of Rochester, hypothesizes that curiosity is a basic component of human nature. He has found that it activates the learning centers of the brain. It is also associated with persistence and problem solving.

Holistic Health

Holistic:

"Rather than focusing on illness or specific parts of the body, this ancient approach to health considers the whole person and how he or she interacts with his or her environment. It emphasizes the connection of mind, body and spirit. The goal is to achieve maximum well-being, where everything is functioning the very best that is possible" (Randall, 2021).

Life Expectancy: Average time a person will live based on gender

Life expectancy changes over the years. As science, technology, and medicine have improved, so has human life expectancy.

Life Span: Maximum amount of time a person can live

In the 17th century, life expectancy numbers were low due to high child and infant mortality. With the inventions of antibiotics and vaccines, these numbers began to improve. Throughout the years science has found ways to extend human life expectancy. One hundred years ago people were expected to live 50–60 years on average. Today our life expectancy has moved to 80 years of age.

Quality of Life (QOL): Referred to as healthy life years (HLY); defined as disability-free life expectancy; distinguishing between years of life free from activity limitations.

Chronic Illness: An illness of long duration that is reoccurring

Acute Illness: Sudden onset and temporary

Occurrences of disability over age 70 tend to center around chronic disease and illnesses such as cardiovascular disease, diabetes, cancer, Alzheimer's, and chronic obstructive pulmonary disease.

Toward a Comprehensive Model for Change

This model for change was developed by Prochaska and DiClemente in 1984 as a plan for changing addictive behavior. The six-step plan can be adapted to fit any plan for change.

Step 1: Precontemplation: What do I want to change?

Step 2: Contemplation: How will I make the changes?

Step 3: Preparation: What resources will I need to be successful? How am I going to make this happen?

Step 4: Action: Getting busy, making a schedule.

Step 5: Maintenance: Stick to your plans. Make notes of hurdles and how you overcame barriers.

Step 6: Termination: If you have succeeded and made this change, there is no need to continue the program.

"Self" Terms

"Self" terms—developing a solid grasp of who we are and where we are going allows for an understanding of "self"

Self-esteem: Confidence in one's own worth or abilities.

Self-concept: A reflection of reactions of others toward ourselves.

Self-efficacy: Belief in one's ability to succeed in specific situations or accomplish specific goals.

References

Life of Wellness. Retrieved April 28, 2021, from https://www.lifeofwelness.ca/

Randall, D. R. (2021, May 19). Claiming Your Wellness. https://ahha.org/helfhelp-articles/claiming-your-wellness/

Prochaska, J.O., James O., John C. Norcross PH.D., and Carlos C. Diclemente PH.D. Changing for Good. New York, NY: HarperCollins Publishers, 1994.

Wang, M. Z., & Hayden, B. Latent Learning, Cognitive Maps, and Curiosity. Curr Opin Behav Sci. 2021 Apr; 38:1–7.

CHAPTER 2

HEALTH CARE

Allopathic Medicine (Western Medicine)

Allopathic Medicine: Traditional Western medicine combating disease with drugs and invasive procedures.

Primary Providers

- **Primary Care Physicians (PCPs):** Personal doctors
- **Nurse Practitioner or Physician's Assistant:** Works with the PCP; can write prescriptions, diagnose, and treat conditions
- **Secondary Care Specialists:** MDs with specialized training

  Examples: Endocrinologist, orthopedic surgeon, oncologist
- **Dentist**
- **Psychiatrist**
- **Pharmacist**

When choosing a health care plan, consumers must be well read on the subject and understand their options. Recognizing your own health care needs and those of your family should dictate the type of medical professional and specialty areas you choose.

As a patient, you must always keep in mind that you are the customer and your doctors and their staffs are providing a service for you.

When seeing a doctor for the first time, come prepared. Create a list of questions beforehand. It is common for people to feel intimidated when they go to the doctor's office. Your list should include any ongoing symptoms or problems that don't go away with over-the-counter treatment.

Knowing Your Numbers (Heo et al., 2021)

Heart Rate: Counting the number of heartbeats per minute. Average = 70 bpm

Blood Pressure: How hard your heart is working. Average = 120/80

Cholesterol: The amount of this dietary fat found in the blood per deciliter of blood (mg/dL). Healthy levels are below 200

Triglycerides: Amount of this dietary fat found in the blood per deciliter of blood. Average should be below 150mg/dL

Fasting Blood Glucose: The amount of sugar (glucose) found in the blood. Good levels are below 100 mg/dL

Body Temperature: The average temperature of the human body is 98.6 degrees

Body Mass Index (BMI): Good levels are 18.5–24.9 kg/m^2

Common Chronic Diseases

- High blood pressure
- High cholesterol
- Arthritis
- Asthma
- Chronic obstructive pulmonary disease
- Inflammatory bowel disease
- Hepatitis C
- Diabetes
- Depression
- Anxiety
- Ischemic heart disease
- Alzheimer's

Ongoing Symptoms That Warrant Concern

- Reoccurring headaches
- Joint aches and pains (with no explanation)
- Digestive abnormalities (chronic diarrhea, cramping, frequent urination)
- Lethargy
- Insomnia
- Ongoing heartburn

Occurrence of these symptoms for more than 2 weeks warrants a trip to your primary care doctor.

The number one cause of death for adults in the United States is cardiovascular disease (CVD).

The second leading cause of death nationwide is cancer (Thomas, 2019).

Osteopathic Medicine: A combination of allopathic medicine and the philosophy that the body has the ability to heal itself

Homeopathic Medicine: A medical system that treats the person as a whole rather than focusing on disease or sickness; it follows the beliefs that "like cures like," there is a single remedy to what ails us, and the minimum dose is the best course of action

Health Care Plans

- Fee for service—pay as you go
- Health Maintenance Organization (HMO)
- Preferred Provider Organization (PPO)
- Student health care—usually provided by colleges and universities; fees are built into admission costs
- Point of Service (POS) plans
- Government insurance options:
  1. Affordable Care Act (ACA), previously called "ObamaCare" and enacted in 2017. Today, over 23 million people are currently covered by this insurance plan (CMS.gov).
  2. Medicare for seniors
  3. Medicaid for low-income individuals
  4. Children's Health Insurance Program (CHIP)

References

CMS.gov. "CMS Fast Facts." CMS. Accessed April 24, 2021. Retrieved October 10, 2020, from https://www.cms.gov/Research-Statistics-Data-and-Systems/Statistics-Trends-and-Reports/CMS-Fast-Facts

Heo, J. (2021). "Four Health Numbers You Should Know." Retrieved October 10, 2020, from https://www.sutterhealth.org/health/heart/four-health-numbers-you-should-know

Thomas, J., & Fraga, J. (2019, September 6). "Causes of Mortality: Our Perceptions vs. Reality." Healthline. Retrieved October 10, 2020, from https://www.healthline.com/health/causes-of-mortality

PHYSICAL HEALTH

CHAPTER 3

FITNESS

Physical Activity: All the day-to-day movement

Physical Fitness: One's ability to exercise at moderate-to-vigorous levels on a regular basis without great fatigue

Exercise: Physical activity carried out for the sake of health and fitness; deliberate movement

> *The Centers for Disease Control and Prevention (CDC, 2021) has found that 80% of American adults do not get the recommended amount of exercise on a daily scale.*
>
> *This equals strength training at least 3 times per week for 30 minutes and moderate-intensity aerobic activity for 2 and a half hours per week.*

Five Components of Fitness

Cardiorespiratory Fitness—exercise that can be maintained over time (longer than 20 minutes without stopping); aerobic (with oxygen).

Muscular Endurance—requires a specific muscle group to sustain activity over a period of time or for a specific number of repetitions. Isokinetic Activity—continuous movement.

Muscular Strength—measured with the movement of a maximum amount of weight one time; anaerobic (without oxygen).

- Can be improved through isotonic movement: moving weight through space for a given number of repetitions and sets; or
- Can be improved through isometric movement: applying pressure to an immovable object

Flexibility—the ability to move a joint through its full range of motion (ROM).

Body Composition—the various tissues that make up the human body; these include fat (adipose) tissue. Lean mass includes muscle tissue, organs, bones, and fluids. Tests measure the percentage of body fat versus lean mass.

A comprehensive exercise program should cover each of the components above. As you commit to your exercise regimen, you may find that it begins to get easier. This would be the time to look at your workouts and determine if you can change one or more aspects.

Following the principle of FITT can guide you in this area.

F = Frequency—How often are you exercising?

I = Intensity—How hard are you pushing yourself?

T = Time—How long are your workouts?

T = Type—Looking at new or different activities to reach your goals.

Benefits of Fitness

Improving your fitness levels will affect every aspect of your life. You will feel more energized, resist disease better, and have an overall improved perceived quality of life.

Improved heart function, stronger muscles, better sleep, and more efficient metabolism, as well as improved mental health, better stress management, and an improved self-image are just some of the many benefits of fitness (Klavora, 2018, p. 238).

Measuring Fitness

Cardiovascular Fitness

Target Heart Range (THR)

Using the personal information of your age and your resting heart rate (RHR), follow the equation below to establish a workout range of heartbeats per minute while you are engaging in cardiovascular exercise.

220 − your age = _____ maximum heart rate (MHR)

MHR − your resting heart rate (RHR) = _____ working heart rate (WHR)

Now establish a range below 100% of your MHR that will provide you the best cardio workout for your fitness level.

WHR × 70% = _____ + RHR = _____ low end of THR

WHR × 85% = _____ + RHR = _____ high end of THR

- 12-minute run

Muscular Endurance

- Timed sit-ups: Count the number of full sit-ups completed in one minute
- Push-up test: Count the number of push-ups that can be completed until fatigue

Muscular Strength

- One repetition, maximum weight

Flexibility

- Hamstring flexibility test
- Sit and reach

References

Azar, A. M. (2019). *Physical Activity Guidelines for Americans*, 2nd ed. Retrieved June 3, 2021, from https:www.cdc.gov/physicalactivity/basics/pa-health/index.htm

Klavora, P. (2018). *Scientific Foundations of Kinesiology: Studying Human Movement and Health*. Kinesiology Books.

CHAPTER 4

NUTRITION

Nutrition: The science of food and its relation to maintenance, growth, reproduction, health, and disease of all organisms

Digestion: A body's ability to break down food into molecules that can be absorbed

Metabolism: The chemical reactions involved in maintaining life

Two types of metabolism:

Catabolism—breakdown of food molecules

Anabolism—the synthesis of the compounds needed by the cells

There are seven major elements of nutrition in the human diet. Three contain calories and four do not. A balanced diet should provide adequate amounts of all seven of these elements.

Calorie: Unit of energy; amount of energy needed to raise the temperature of 1 gram of water by 1 degree

Empty Calorie: Sugars, fats, oils, and alcohol provide calories with no nutrient value

Dietary Elements That Contain Calories

Macronutrients

Carbohydrates: <u>All carbohydrates contain 4 calories per gram</u>. This dietary element is the body's preferred form of energy and is broken down into three groups: simple sugars, complex carbohydrates, and fiber.

Simple sugars and complex carbohydrates are broken down into glycogen. Fiber does not break down and passes through the intestinal tract.

Simple sugars are easily broken down by the body and provide quick surges in energy levels.

Complex carbohydrates are longer-lasting forms of energy, taking up to 24 hours to digest.

Fiber: Plant based nutrients containing roughage. Soluble fiber increases fullness and slows digestion. It can help lose fat and prevent belly fat. Adding just 10 grams of soluble fiber to your diet can lower your risk of belly fat gain.

Insoluble fiber passes through the digestive system, providing bulk to digestive waste.

Fats (Lipids): All fats contain 9 calories per gram. This dietary element is used for backup energy and is necessary for the following bodily functions: insulating and cushioning vital organs; absorption of fat-soluble vitamins; and the synthesis of sex hormones.

Fats that should be avoided or consumed in moderation:

Saturated Fats—generally solid at room temperature. These types of fats are very difficult for the body to break down. Chemically, fats are made up of hydrogen and carbon. These molecules have *carbon bonds that are saturated with hydrogen.*

Cholesterol—a fatlike, waxy material found in animal products and produced by the body.

Trans Fats (TFAs)—naturally occurring in some foods; most trans fats are made from oils through a food processing method called hydrogenation (partial hydrogenation).

Healthy Fats
Monounsaturated fats have one carbon bond missing a hydrogen bond, making it easier to break down. Food examples include nuts, avocado, canola, and sesame and olive oils.

Polyunsaturated fats have more than one carbon bond without hydrogen, making it easier to break down. Food examples include walnuts, sunflower seeds, flax, "fishy" fish, safflower, and corn and soybean oils.

Triglycerides—make up most of the fat you eat. When you eat these fats, your body converts calories it doesn't need to use right away into triglycerides. These are stored in fat cells. Later, your body will release these for energy between meals.

What leads to high levels of triglycerides? Obesity, regular alcohol use, uncontrolled diabetes, and a high-calorie diet.

Proteins
All proteins have 4 calories per gram and are the main tissue builders for every cell. They are found in meat, dairy, nuts, and some grains and beans.

Amino Acids—These are left after proteins are digested and broken down. Of the 20 amino acids, 9 are essential, meaning that they must be gotten from the diet. The remaining 11 are nonessential, meaning that the body produces them. These components break down food, help with growth, and repair body tissue.

Micronutrients

Fiber—a carbohydrate that does not break down completely. These substances move through the digestive tract, taking debris with it. Fiber is necessary for a healthy digestive tract.

Minerals—inorganic substances that regulate and play an important role in growth, bone health, and fluid balance. There are 13 minerals that are essential and when not adequately consumed can cause specific deficiency symptoms. These minerals include sodium, iron, iodine, potassium, zinc, magnesium, manganese, calcium, fluoride, phosphorous, selenium, chloride, and copper (Health Information from the National Library of Medicine, 2021).

Vitamins—organic substances that must be gotten from our diets. These are necessary for energy production, immune function, and blood clotting.

Water-soluble vitamins can be flushed from the system if taken in too great a quantity. These include vitamin C and B vitamins, including thiamine (B1), riboflavin (B2), niacin (B3), pantothenic acid (B5), pyridoxine (B6), biotin (B7), folate (B9), and cobalamin (B12).

Fat-soluble vitamins are stored in the fat tissue and can collect to the point of toxicity. These include vitamins A, D, E, and K.

Water—approximately 60% of the human body is water. Standard recommended consumption is 3 liters of water per day.

Toxicity—too much of a substance

Deficiency—not enough of a substance

Other Dietary Issues and Concerns

Phytonutrients (antioxidants) are compounds produced by plants that keep them healthy, protecting them from insects and the sun. These compounds are found in colorful fruits and vegetables, whole grains, tea, beans, spices, and nuts. They possess an anti-inflammatory agent beneficial to the body. They also neutralize free radicals. Benefits of some phytonutrients include:

- *Carotenoids*—for eye health
- *Resveratrol*—for cognitive health
- *Flavonoids*—cancer fighters
- *Phytoestrogens*—heart health

Free Radicals: Natural by-products of metabolism. These are activated oxygen ions with an uneven number of electrons. These unstable atoms attack healthy cells and steal their electrons, making them dysfunctional. This damage causes illness and aging.

Genetically Modified Organisms (GMOs): Any organism whose genetic material has been altered using genetic engineering techniques. Genetic engineering is a lab process where genes of one species are removed and artificially forced into the genes of an unrelated plant or animal.

Organic Foods: Meats, fruits, and vegetables that are free from synthetic herbicides, pesticides, or fertilizer. The same guidelines apply to animal food products as well as ensuring that the animals are not fed antibiotics or hormones. Hens must be uncaged and have outdoor access, and cows must go to pasture at least 120 days a year. These are guidelines recommended by FACT (Food Animal Concerns Trust) and required for a USDA Organic stamp of approval.

Inflammation: A process in the body where body tissues and organs become swollen due to the buildup of white blood cells and other blood products. This response is often triggered by outside agents. Certain food types can cause a deadly reaction in some people.

Glycemic Index: This chart provides numbers for carbohydrates based on how fast your body converts them to glucose (blood sugar). The higher the number, the more quickly your body breaks down these foods. A score of 55 or less is considered low, while a score over 70 indicates a faster metabolization.

Glucose: The body's preferred source of energy gotten from foods.

Food Intolerance: Certain foods cause an adverse reaction when consumed by some people. Symptoms include diarrhea, bloating, rash, headaches, nausea, fatigue, reflux, abdominal pain, and runny nose. The most common foods causing these reactions include, but are not limited to:

> gluten, shellfish, peanuts, dairy, caffeine, alcohol, sugars, and monosodium glutamate (MSG).

Food Desert: Any community that doesn't have access to fresh produce and proteins within a mile of their residence.

Dietary Types

Vegetarian: Exclusion of meat or other animal products from the diet

> *Ovo*—eggs, but no dairy

> *Lacto*—dairy, but no eggs

> *Pesca*—no meats, just fish

Vegan: No meat or animal products

> *Raw Vegan*—vegan, but no vegetables cooked above 48°C

Diet: A temporary food consumption plan designed for weight loss

> Evaluate the strengths and weaknesses of your diet. Ask yourself:
> 1. Is my diet nutritionally balanced?

2. How often do I eat throughout the day?
3. Do I stay hydrated?
4. Am I eating after 9 PM?
5. Do I skip a morning meal?

Reference

Health Information from the National Library for Medicine, MedlinePlus. (2021, April 28). U.S. National Library of Medicine. https://medlineplus.gov/

CHAPTER 5

WEIGHT MANAGEMENT

WEIGHT MANAGEMENT IS AN ONGOING CONCERN for the majority of Americans. Whether it is the need to lose weight, gain weight, or maintain a healthy weight, it is a major factor for an overall healthy life. Those who want to make a significant change in their weight must begin by addressing these three areas:

Evaluating weaknesses and strengths of current dietary choices (see Chapter 4):

- Cutting down on high-fat, high-calorie foods
- Eating four to six times a day in small servings
- Hydration

Physical activity and exercise (see Chapter 3):

- Physical activity: take the stairs, choose to walk
- Exercise 5 to 6 hours per week

Identifying behaviors that are counterproductive to your goals, behavior modification. Making changes to assist in achieving your weight management goals.

- Don't skip breakfast; consume healthy calories within 1 hour of waking
- Portion control
- Eliminate late-night eating or eat healthy, low-calorie foods after 8:00 PM.

Body Composition

Essential Body Fat: Fat necessary for your body to perform the following: provide cushioning and insulation for vital organs; completion of cellular structure; absorption of fat-soluble vitamins; and synthesis of sex hormones

Men—no less than 5%   Women—no less than 12%

Nonessential Body Fat: All other fat found on the body

Subcutaneous—fat found just below the skin and above muscle tissue

Visceral—surrounding organs

Lean Body Mass: A large portion of total body weight comes from lean mass. This includes muscle, organs, and bone

Obesity in America

In 2021, approximately 42.5% of US adults over the age of 20 were found to be obese (Fryar et al., 2021). Obesity is a health issue affecting many Americans. There are many causes for this problem, including genetic predisposition, poor nutrition behaviors, medication use, and environment.

The consequences of obesity are many. It is directly linked to life-threatening diseases such as diabetes, cardiovascular disease, stroke, and some types of cancer.

Obese vs. Overweight

Obese: 42.5% of US adults aged 20 and over have obesity, including 9% classified as severely obese

Morbid Obesity—40% body fat. Body fat is directly related to some diseases that can be life threatening.

Overweight—weighing too much according to height/weight charts (Fryar et al., 2021).

Body Fat Testing

Height/Weight Charts

Body Mass Index (BMI) Using Gender, Height, and Weight

Skin Calipers: Measure skin folds (subcutaneous) at specific sites on the body, most commonly hip, back, arm, thigh, and abdomen.

Hydrostatic Tank: Compares body weight outside the water to body weight when completely submerged. Using these numbers and the density of the water, the subject's body density can be accurately calculated. This number is used to estimate total body composition.

Bioelectrical Impedance: Two sets of electrodes are attached to the subject's left foot and left hand. Personal information is typed into the computer, and then an electrical impulse is sent through the body, measuring how quickly these impulses return.

Dual-Energy X-ray Absorptiometry (DEXA): Originally used for bone density testing, the DEXA has proven to be very efficient in measuring total body composition.

Bod-Pod Air-Displacement Plethysmography: The Bod-Pod acts along the same principles as hydrostatic weighing, but instead of using water, it uses the displacement of air and the overall mass of the body.

Health Risks Associated with Obesity

Diabetes

High blood pressure

Cardiovascular disease

Cancers

Arthritis

Weight Management Principles

Dieting: Diet implies temporary weight loss. Once you go off a diet, you must modify your eating habits in order to avoid regaining the lost weight: 75% of people who go on a diet return to their old habits of eating and regain their weight. This is called yo-yo dieting.

Fasting: Abstaining from calorie consumption for a set amount of time. While medical and religious fasting is well regulated, most fasts are self-regulated. Those who embark on fasts for weight loss must be very careful that they do not deny their bodies' need for certain nutrients and stay hydrated.

Managing Metabolism: Metabolism is the way the human body burns calories from the food we consume. We convert these calories into energy to assist in all physical functions.

The following are seven behaviors one must engage in to successfully manage one's metabolism.

- *Balance:* Eat an equal share of all food components.
- *Nutrient timing:* A University of Massachusetts study found that those who skipped their morning meal were 4.5 times more likely to be overweight than those who didn't.
- *Self-monitoring:* Recognize poor nutritional choices and eliminate them.
- *Selective restrictions:* Cut back on high-calorie foods, but avoid being punitive in your restrictions.
- *Calorie counting:* Make note of daily calorie consumption, keeping intake around the same amount. Portion control is important.
- *Consistency in consumption:* Avoid getting hungry, which assists in metabolism regulation.

- *Motivation:* Stick to a program and follow through to achieve goals.

Energy balance equation: Calories consumed – calories burned during activity = weight

Fat Cell Theory: Fat cell development is unique in every human being. The body typically develops fat cells in utero, during the first year of life, and through puberty. After these periods, fat cells will only appear if the body is forced to find room for excessive ingestion of fat calories.

Genetic Predisposition: Human body types can be genetically predetermined.

Weight Loss Treatment Options

Drugs (Synthetic): These are all prescription drugs. While approved by the FDA, it is recommended that the user stop use if there is no weight loss after 12 weeks.

Some examples of these drugs are:

Xenical—fat burner

Qsymia—a stimulant that suppresses the appetite

Olestra—a "fat binder." When you consume this drug, the body does not digest fat, sending it straight to the large intestine.

Saxenda—a diabetes drug that signals the body that it is full

Surgical: Procedures that alter the digestive anatomy, making caloric absorption more difficult for the body. Suppressing appetite and changing metabolism. Candidates for these surgeries are those with severe obesity (BMI over 30) who have been unsuccessful with traditional weight loss or who suffer from serious health problems caused by their excess weight.

Three types of bariatric surgery most commonly done in the United States:

- *Laparoscopic adjustable gastric band*—A ring with an inner, inflatable band is placed at the top of the stomach, creating a small pouch. This pouch is much smaller than the stomach and fills up faster, causing feelings of fullness. The band can be adjusted by the surgeon. Once weight loss has been achieved, it can be removed.

- *Gastric sleeve (vertical sleeve gastrectomy)*—This surgery removes most of the stomach, leaving a banana-shaped section that is closed with staples. The rest of the stomach is removed. The stomach is smaller so you get full faster. Taking out part of the stomach also affects gut hormones and gut bacteria. This is not reversible.

- *Gastric bypass (Roux-en-Y gastric bypass)*—The surgeon staples the stomach, leaving a small pouch in the upper section. Next, the surgeon cuts the small intestine and attaches the lower part of it directly to the small stomach pouch. Food bypasses most of the stomach and the upper part of the small intestine, so the body absorbs fewer calories. The bypassed section is attached farther down to the lower part of the small intestine. This allows digestive juices from the stomach to move into that lower section, facilitating digestion. Since nothing is removed, it can be reversed with some difficulty.

After these surgeries the patient is given supplements to make sure they are getting adequate amounts of vitamins and minerals. Physical activity is encouraged, with care. For the first few weeks your diet is strictly monitored, beginning with a liquid diet, then soft foods (cottage cheese, yogurt, and soup), then solid foods. Small meals and chewing your food well are important. Weight loss will vary from person to person and will take time. A study following patients for 3 years after surgery found that they lost about 45 lbs. with the band and 90 lbs. with the bypass.

vBloc Therapy: Controlled electrical stimulation that stimulates the brain to recognize that you are not hungry.

Aspire Assist: A device much like a feeding tube is inserted into the stomach and is used to empty the stomach after eating before the majority of digestion occurs.

Liposuction (Lipoplasty or Body Contouring): Using a suction technique, the doctor removes fat from specific areas of the body, usually the abdomen, hips, thighs, buttocks, arms, or neck. Does not remove cellulite.

Cellulite: Fat beneath the skin that causes a lumpy look.

Eating Disorders

According to ANAD.org (2021):

- At least 30 million people in the United States suffer from an eating disorder.
- Every 62 minutes at least one person dies as a direct result of an eating disorder.
- Eating disorders have the highest mortality rate of any mental illness.

Anorexia Nervosa: An eating disorder characterized by weight loss; a distorted body image; and trouble maintaining appropriate weight for height, age, and gender. This is a life-threatening disorder.

Bulimia Nervosa: A cycle of binge eating and purging or heavy laxative use; considered a mental illness if these behaviors continue at least one time per week for 12 weeks.

Binge Eating Disorder (BED): Eating large amounts of food quickly and to the point of discomfort; a feeling of loss of control during the binge, experiencing shame, guilt, or distress afterward. There is no purging or behavior to counter the excessive food ingestion.

Pica: Eating nonfood items such as dirt, paint chips, hair, or chalk.

Orthorexia: Obsession with "proper" eating.

Diabulimia: Improper use of insulin replacement drugs for weight loss.

References

Eating Disorder Statistics: General & Diversity Stats: ANAD. National Association of Anorexia Nervosa and Associated
Disorders. (2021, March 3). https://anad.org/get-informed/about-eating-disorders/eating-disorders-statistics/

Fryar, C. D., Carroll, M. D., & Afful, J. (2021, January 29). Prevalence of overweight, obesity, and severe obesity among
adults aged 20 and over: United States, 1060–1062 through 2017–2018. https://www.cdc.gov/nchs/datal/hestat/
obesity-adult-17-18/obesity-htm

MENTAL HEALTH, ILLNESS, AND ADDICTION

CHAPTER 6

STRESS AND MENTAL HEALTH

S TRESS IS A HUMAN CONDITION THAT was researched and defined in the early 1930s by Dr. Hans Selye.

Stress: The nonspecific response of the body to any demand made upon it.

> *Eustress*—life experiences that are positive

> *Distress*—life experiences that are negative

> *Stressor*—an agent that elicits the stress response

The Stress of Life (1956) by Hans Selye explains his General Adaptation Syndrome (GAS). This book discusses the living organism's response to stress and what happens over time as stress builds up.

Broken down into three stages, the stress response relies on recognition of the stressor. This recognition occurs in the first stage.

Stages of the General Adaptation Syndrome (GAS)

Alarm: As the stressor is recognized, there is a short burst of energy necessary for a reaction.

Resistance: Once recognized, the organism enters the "fight-or-flight" mode. Here, there is a split-second decision made whether to engage with the stressor or to flee.

Exhaustion: If the stressor is more powerful or able to overcome the person under stress, then there is defeat.

Physiological response to stress: When under stress, the body goes through the following signs or symptoms: sweating, high blood pressure, increase in heart rate, increased respiration, heightened alertness, and the release of the hormones adrenaline, noradrenaline, cortisol, and epinephrine.

Stress Management

Time management

Fiscal responsibility

Gratitude

Exercise

Mindfulness

Positive nutritional habits

Journaling

Personality Types

Type A—assertive, timely, attention to detail

Type B—easygoing, laid back

Defense Mechanisms

In the short term, strategies used to help get through a difficult situation can be helpful coping mechanisms, but they are not considered good long-term healthy behaviors.

There are three categories of defense mechanisms identified by the American Psychiatric Association (APA): primitive, less primitive, and mature. I have included two examples from each category.

<u>Primitive:</u> Less likely to be effective in the short term.

- *Denial*—refusal to accept reality
- *Projection*—putting your thoughts, feelings, or impulses onto another person who doesn't have these thoughts. Blaming them for your inadequacies.

<u>Less Primitive:</u> Not ideal ways of dealing with stress.

- *Intellectualization*—overemphasizing thinking in order to distance yourself from the unwanted impulse, behavior, or event
- *Rationalization*—putting something in a different light or offering other explanations that are not reality based

<u>Mature:</u> Most constructive and helpful. These can be healthy reactions to difficult situations.

- *Compensation*—counterbalancing perceived weaknesses by emphasizing strengths in other areas
- *Assertiveness*—emphasizing your needs in a way that is respectful, direct, and firm

Maslow's Hierarchy of Needs

In 1954 Abraham Maslow created a hierarchy listing human needs in order of necessity. The needs begin at the base, recognizing that humans have basic survival needs that supersede all other needs. This is typically portrayed in a pyramid (McLeod, 2020).

Level 1—Physiological needs—food, water, sleep, and sex

Level 2—Safety needs—shelter and security

Level 3—Love and belonging

Level 4—Self-esteem

Level 5—Self-actualization

References

McLeod, S. (2020). Maslow's Hierarchy of Needs. Simply Psychology. https://www.simplypsychology.org/maslow.html

Selye, H. (1956). *The Stress of Life*. McGraw-Hill.

CHAPTER 7

MENTAL ILLNESS

THE AMERICAN PSYCHIATRIC ASSOCIATION (APA) IDENTIFIES mental illnesses by their signs and symptoms in its text, *The Diagnostic and Statistical Manual* (DSM). Every 10 years, this book is updated. In 2022 the DSM-V is the current updated version. The mental illnesses discussed in this chapter are listed in this edition.

The top seven mental illnesses in college students are: anxiety, depression, addiction, ADHD (attention deficit hyperactive disorder), bipolar disorder, and PTSD (post-traumatic stress disorder). According to a survey of college counseling center directors, the number of students with significant psychological problems is growing. Anxiety is the top concern.

Depression

Depression is a mental illness that affects how you feel, think, and behave, causing persistent feelings of sadness and loss of interest in previously enjoyed activities.

Considered clinical if symptoms persist for more than 6 weeks.

Mild depression—not seriously debilitating; manifests as sadness, lack of interest in things you once enjoyed, and lethargy that lasts for more than 6 weeks

Major depressive disorder—severe and disabling to the point of impaired function. No longer engaging in daily routines, avoiding social situations, and sleeping or eating too much or too little. Suicidal thoughts may also be present.

Depression and grief: What is the difference?

The APA has included "bereavement exclusion" when diagnosing depression, noting that major depression should not be diagnosed in individuals within the first 2 months following the death of a loved one.

Grief—painful feelings that come in waves (after a loss) and are intermixed with positive memories. Self-esteem stays intact.

Depression—same feelings due to loss, but interest and pleasure are decreased for a minimum of 2 weeks. Behavior changes include a lack of interest in activities once enjoyed, no social motivation, and self-medication with mind-altering substances to the point of abuse. Feelings of self-loathing and worthlessness.

When grief and depression coexist, the grief lasts longer and the effects are more intense.

Bipolar disorder—severe mood swings of depression and manic behavior with lulls between episodes. Some people experience remission where they are symptom free. It is important to treat this disease regardless of where someone is in their cycle, as the depressive mood swings can be severe and lead to suicide.

While depression is more pervasive, mania can cause more problems in one's family life, work, and friendships. Mania is a mix of irritability, anger, and euphoria. This elation may manifest as overconfidence playing out in bouts of overcommitting, overspending, or promiscuity.

Suicide: The taking of one's own life. No one knows where these impulses to take our own lives begin. Are they sudden impulses or prolonged? What is clear is that suicide is NOT something that the survivors can predict or take blame for.

It is the second leading cause of death among 15- to 24-year-olds in the United States and the tenth leading cause of death overall. Access to a gun triples the risk of suicide.

"... it is very likely that once suicide occurred and others were cognizant of it, the act was repeated ... in part because animals and humans learn, to considerable extent, through imitation. Suicide, dangerously, has a contagious aspect; it has, as well, for the vulnerable, an indisputable appeal as the solution of last resort." (Redfield-Jamison, 1999, p. 44)

Anxiety Disorders

Panic Disorder—Sudden and repeated episodes of intense fear accompanied by physical symptoms such as chest pain, rapid heartbeat, trouble catching your breath, vertigo, and gastrointestinal problems. Women are two times more likely to suffer from panic disorder than men.

Phobias—Irrational and disabling fears. People with phobias will do anything to avoid what they are afraid of. Some life events can trigger this fear. A car accident causes you to avoid cars, a dog bite causes fear of all dogs, etc.

- Agoraphobia—the most common phobia in the United States. Fears include leaving your home, large crowds, and feelings of being trapped.

- Social Anxiety Disorder—social phobia causing overwhelming fear of situations that require interacting with other people or performing in front of others. This also includes a fear that you may humiliate yourself with your actions while in public.

General Anxiety Disorder (GAD): One of the most common anxiety disorders, this condition manifests in uncontrollable worry. Regardless of the situation, sufferers experience an inability to concentrate due to their feelings of pending doom.

Seasonal Affective Disorder (SAD): Symptoms include sleepiness, trouble concentrating, carbohydrate cravings, lethargy, weight gain, and decreased libido. Most commonly occurs in geographical areas where there is not a lot of sunshine or for people who work nights and sleep throughout the day.

Post-traumatic Stress Syndrome/Disorder (PTSS/PTSD): A disorder caused by a terrifying event. Reminders of these events trigger symptoms. These symptoms include flashbacks, nightmares, severe anxiety, and uncontrolled thoughts of the event.

Obsessive-Compulsive and Related Disorders (OCRD)

Created as a new category of mental illness, these conditions all have an obsessive-compulsive behavior within the overall signs and symptoms.

Obsessive-Compulsive Disorder: Repetitive thoughts accompanied by ritualistic behaviors.

Hoarding: Excessive saving of items others may view as worthless. This can lead to clutter that disrupts one's ability to live in a healthy environment.

Body Dysmorphic Disorder: Obsession with real or perceived body flaws that cause severe distress and problems with daily functioning. The sufferer focuses on his or her imperfections to the point of distraction.

Eating Disorders: As discussed in Chapter 5, these disorders surround food. The sufferer uses food as a distraction from situations that cause anxiety.

Attention Deficit/Hyperactivity Disorder (ADHD)

A disorder that begins in childhood and continues into adulthood. Characterized by a pattern of behaviors, present in multiple settings (school, home, etc.) that can result in performance issues. Broken down into two categories (inattention hyperactivity and impulsivity), behaviors such as failure to pay close attention to detail, difficulty organizing tasks and activities, excessive talking, fidgeting, or an inability to remain seated.

Personality Disorders

Abnormal, ingrained patterns of behavior that deviate from social norms; trouble with interpersonal skills, impulse control, and cognition. Individuals with personality disorders pay excessive attention to detail, resulting in poor work/life balance. They can be rigid and stubborn as well as preoccupied with tasks. There are 10 distinct types of personality disorders:

Paranoid; schizoid; schizotypal; antisocial; borderline; histrionic; dependent; narcissistic; avoidant; and obsessive-compulsive (DSM-V).

Dissociative Identity Disorder

Multiple personality disorder. This person's identities are fragmented into two or more personality states. Generally linked to those who have suffered extreme abuse, especially in childhood.

Neurosis vs. Psychosis

- A neurotic person presents as overanxious, oversensitive, or obsessive to the point that it causes distress in the form of depression or anxiety. This person is still in touch with reality.

- A psychotic person is NOT in touch with reality; their behavior is unpredictable and odd. Psychosis may include hallucinations and delusions.

Schizophrenia

Schizophrenia is an incurable mental illness that manifests in different types of behaviors and actions. Approximately 1% of the population in the United States is schizophrenic. Depending on the type or types one suffers from, the symptoms can vary and overlap. The onset of schizophrenia usually occurs in one's late teens or early 20s.

Drug-induced onset can occur at any age if you have a genetic history of the disease and have abused illicit stimulants (crack, meth, etc.).

The most common symptoms of schizophrenia include the following:

Psychosis	Disorganized speech
Hallucinations	Strange or odd behavior
Delusions	Paranoia

Types of schizophrenia include the following:

- Paranoid

- Disorganized—speech and thoughts

- Residual—symptoms that remain after treatment

- Schizoaffective—any of the above with a dual diagnosis of bipolar disorder

- Schizophreniform—early onset, beginning in childhood. Symptoms seem to be less severe

- Catatonic—lifeless, withdrawn; this person is usually institutionalized

Addiction

As discussed in Chapter 8, addiction is a brain disorder characterized by the compulsive use of drugs or engagement in behaviors perceived as rewarding. The continuation of this behavior gives the user a feeling of euphoria, promoting continued use or participation.

References

Redfield-Jamison, K. (1999). *Night Falls Fast: Understanding Suicide*. Alfred A. Knopf. https://www.randomhouse.com

Zimmerman, Mark. Overview of Personality Disorders. May 2021. www.merckmanuals.com/professional/psychiatric-disorders/overview-of-personality-disorders

CHAPTER 8

ADDICTION

Addictive Behavior

Addiction: A brain disorder characterized by the compulsive use of stimuli perceived or felt as rewarding. The continuation of this behavior is reinforced by pleasurable feelings (Colon-Rivera, 2020). A treatable chronic medical disease involving complex interactions among brain circuits, genetics, the environment, and an individual's life experiences.

The euphoria felt by an addict is temporary, causing the user to "chase the high."

Behaviors of addiction (sometimes referred to as "maladaptive behaviors") cause those who suffer from this disease to compulsively engage due to perceived reward. This is a difficult problem to tackle due to the stigma associated with substance abuse and addiction.

The most common form of addiction is substance abuse, which may cause any or all of the following:

Impaired Control—cravings to use a substance with desired or failed attempts to control this use

Social Problems—failure to complete major tasks at school, home, or work due to substance use

Risky Use—substance is used in risky situations despite known risk. May also engage in substance use prior to engaging in an activity that requires coordination and stable thought.

Drug Effects/Tolerance—escalation and withdrawal are present.

    Tolerance—the physiological desire for higher doses

    Escalation—the behaviors engaged in to get the higher dosage

Enabler: One who removes the consequences of someone's negative behaviors by making excuses or ignoring the behavior altogether. Enablers make it easier for the addict to engage in their drug use (Colon-Rivera, 2020).

Drug Effects

Therapeutic levels—recommended dosage for specific conditions

Synergism—when two or more drugs are taken and the effects are intensified

Polydrug Use—using more than one drug at a time

Drug Expectancy—knowing how a drug will affect you; taking into consideration your SET (state of mind) and SETTING (your environment)

Drug Use

Drug Use—using a drug for the condition it was meant to treat and in the recommended dosage

Drug Misuse—using a drug for the condition it was meant to treat but in a greater dosage than recommended

Drug Abuse—using a drug recreationally. Not prescribed, and dosage is not adhered to

Alcohol

Ethanol is a fossil fuel and the type of alcohol produced by brewing, fermenting, and distilling fruits, vegetables, and grains. When digested, it is changed by the body into acetaldehyde, which is a poison in the human body and a close relative of formaldehyde, used for embalming.

The legal age to purchase and consume alcohol in the United States is 21. The blood alcohol concentration (BAC) legal limit is 0.08 grams per ml of blood.

Proof value vs. percent of alcohol—the proof value is a number created by the makers of alcoholic products to enhance sales. The proof value number reflects twice the actual percentage of alcohol in their product. For example, something that is 100 proof has 50% alcohol in it.

One drink is the equivalent of 12 oz. of beer, 5 oz. of wine, or 1.5 oz. of spirits.

Physiological Effects of Alcohol

Metabolizing Alcohol: The liver is the primary site (80%) in the human body for the metabolism of alcohol. The body breaks down alcohol in a similar manner as it does with fat. The resulting product of metabolized alcohol is fatty acids. Alcohol contributes 7 calories per gram to the human diet. The remaining 20% of the alcohol is broken down in the pancreas and gastrointestinal tract.

Absorption of Alcohol: While we begin alcohol absorption in the oral cavity, the majority is absorbed in the small intestine. As it is absorbed through the intestinal walls, it is released into the blood stream, where it makes its way to the brain, affecting the central nervous system. In low concentrations, alcohol reduces inhibitions and gives the user a feeling of euphoria. While these levels climb, behavior goes from mild euphoria to impaired sensory and motor coordination and eventually to mental confusion.

Mothers Against Drunk Driving (MADD)

Founded in 1980 by a mother who lost her son to a drunk driver, MADD is an advocacy group fighting against drunk driving. It supports the victims of drunk driving and those families and friends who have lost a loved one to a drunk driver.

Driving Under the Influence (DUI)—legal violation determined by law enforcement in the field. Violation can lead to loss of license, community service, forced attendance at drug/alcohol recovery meetings, and financial fines.

- Drunk driving impacts two in three people across the country.
- One person is killed every 50 minutes in an alcohol-related auto accident in the United States.

Alcohol Dependence—a chronic disease in which a person craves alcohol and is unable to control their drinking. Someone who is dependent on alcohol cannot stop drinking without experiencing painful effects. Quitting "cold turkey" can be fatal.

Problem drinker: A person who has difficulty in their life as a result of their alcohol use. They may not have developed full-blown alcoholism yet but are on their way.

Heavy drinker: Defined as 15 drinks per week for men and 8 drinks per week for women. People who engage in this behavior die, on average, 24 to 28 years earlier than those who do not drink.

Binge drinker: Periodic drinking. Bingers can go weeks without drinking, but when they do drink they drink to drunkenness. Defined as drinking 4 to 5 drinks within a 2-hour span.

Alcoholism: A chronic disease characterized by uncontrolled drinking and a preoccupation with alcohol. This individual has lost the ability to control their drinking. This condition is recognized as a chronic illness by the American Medical Association and a chronic mental illness by the American Psychiatric Association.

Alcohol and Health Concerns

Cardiovascular Disease: High blood pressure, arrhythmia, coronary artery disease, cardiomyopathy, congestive heart failure

Liver: Cirrhosis

Cancers: Oral, esophageal, small and large intestine, colon, pancreas, liver, kidneys

Alcohol Addiction Recovery

Alcohol withdrawal is the most dangerous type of withdrawal from an addictive substance. Symptoms include seizures, tremors, increased respiration, increased heart rate, nausea, insomnia, and hallucinations. Delirium tremens (DT) is another symptom of alcohol withdrawal. Symptoms include confusion, irritability, seizures, and hallucinations. This condition can be fatal.

Most patients require some type of inpatient care during detoxification from alcohol.

Alcohol detoxification is an inpatient treatment that is the alcoholic's first step to "getting clean." It may take up to 5 days (sometimes longer). While in treatment, the alcoholic is given drugs that block the symptoms of withdrawal and ease the discomfort caused by the lack of alcohol in the system. According to the National Institute of Alcohol Abuse and Alcoholism (NIAAA), approximately 17 million Americans currently have Alcohol Use Disorder (AUD).

Tobacco

Tobacco is an organic substance that is harvested, dried, and processed mostly for its recreational use. There are three major components in processed tobacco:

Nicotine—the addictive agent in tobacco

Tar—the particulate matter found in tobacco smoke. This is a carcinogen.

Carbon monoxide—a chemical that displaces oxygen in the smoker's blood

There are thousands of damaging chemicals found in tobacco smoke. Most of these products are damaging and poisonous to the human body. From arsenic to zinc, the list is long, and the reasons for the presence of these substances are vague. Some occur naturally in tobacco, and some are added to the product during processing.

Forms of Tobacco

Cigarettes: Processed tobacco rolled in paper with a filter attached to one end

Cigars and Pipes: Similar to cigarettes, but most smokers do not inhale the smoke

Bidis: Small, hand rolled cigarettes wrapped in an Asian tendu leaf; often flavored

Hookah: Water pipe with one or more hoses, a bowl for tobacco and fruit (for flavor), and mouthpieces. A chamber is filled with water; on the top of the chamber is a bowl where charcoal is lit. Then, tobacco and fruit or other flavoring is also piled into the bowl.

E-cigarettes (Vaping): Flavored vapor smoked out of a device that heats the liquid into a vapor

Smokeless Tobacco: Four ways tobacco is used for its nicotine that don't include combustion. Chewing, snuffing, pinch between cheek and gum, application to skin in the form of patches. The consumer will get more nicotine per dosage from smokeless tobacco than by smoking.

The Smoke

Mainstream (firsthand) smoke: The smoke that is inhaled directly into the smoker's lungs

Side-stream (secondhand) smoke: The environmental smoke inhaled by the nonsmoker

Thirdhand smoke: The residue found in the environment of a smoker

Tobacco and Health Concerns

Cancers: Oral, esophageal, larynx, kidney, bladder, pancreas, cervical, and stomach

Leukemia

Cardiovascular disease: High blood pressure, arrhythmia, anemia, coronary heart disease

Chronic obstructive pulmonary disease (COPD): Chronic bronchitis and emphysema

Macular degeneration: Blindness

Cannabis

The definition for the legal use of marijuana varies from state to state. While many states in the United States have legalized medical marijuana, only a few have legalized its use recreationally.

Marijuana: A depressant, this plant is green and leafy. It is known for its multiple uses in cultures worldwide.

Hemp: Used to make textiles, biofuels, paper, clothing, and rope.

Cannabinoids (CBDs): Oils that relieve aches and pains, working together with the endocannabinoid system of the body. No psychoactive properties.

The psychoactive component in cannabis is tetrahydrocannabinol (THC).

Three strains of psychoactive marijuana used recreationally are:

- Sativa—energizing
- Indica—deep state of relaxation
- Ruderalis—not as psychotropic as the other two

All three stimulate the appetite, relax muscle spasticity, and sedate.

Medical marijuana is used to treat a myriad of conditions and illnesses, including seizures, glaucoma, PTSD, schizophrenia, Alzheimer's, Crohn's, anorexia, multiple sclerosis, side effects from chemotherapy, muscle spasticity, pain, appetite loss, and much more.

Cannabis can be smoked, eaten, applied to the skin, or used in tinctures.

Legal Issues

The laws governing the use of cannabis vary from state to state, but the federal government (under the Controlled Substances Act, CSA) still lists marijuana as a Schedule I drug, meaning that it is recognized as having a high potential for abuse, has no medicinal benefits, and cannot be safely prescribed. It is a federal crime to possess, buy, or sell marijuana.

Even if your state has legalized recreational marijuana use, you may still be penalized for possession. If you are arrested for possession or sales, penalties can be life altering. Some of the areas that may affect your life include:

Employment—You can be fired from your job for testing positive for THC. Doctors can lose their license for prescribing marijuana.

Housing—Renters can be evicted if their lease prohibits illegal drug use on the premises.

Gun Ownership—If you have a medical marijuana card, you can be prevented from buying a gun.

Legal Records—A marijuana possession arrest or misdemeanor will go on one's arrest record, which is a publicly accessible document. Future employers can deny employment based on this information. You can lose the ability to purchase insurance, become ineligible for a mortgage, and be denied student financial aid (Johnston et al., 2015).

Other Psychoactive Drugs

Psychoactive drugs are any substance that, when taken, changes the user's mood or behavior.
Categories:

- Over the counter (OTC)—legal to purchase
- Prescription—can only be gotten with a doctor's prescription
- Illicit—illegal

Stimulants

Sometimes referred to as "uppers," all stimulants are highly addictive. These drugs speed up mental and physical processes, which can produce desirable effects by increasing levels of dopamine in the brain. There are both legal and illegal stimulants, and both categories can lead to addiction.

Legal types of stimulants include caffeine and nicotine.

Betel Nut: A Schedule IV drug (legal by prescription only) in the United States, this substance acts as a stimulant for the user. Usually chewed by the user, this seed of the Areca catechu palm tree is found in Southeast Asia and the Pacific Islands (Guam, the Philippines, etc.).

Cocaine: Made from the leaves of the coca plant, cocaine comes in the form of a white powder. The most common form of ingestion is snorting. Prolonged use may include loss of appetite, sleeplessness, agitation, and hallucinations. This drug is legally used as an anesthetic.

Crack: A derivative of cocaine, it comes in the form of a crystalized rock and is most commonly smoked or injected.

Amphetamine: A prescription drug used to treat ADHD, narcolepsy, and obesity.

Methamphetamine: A Schedule II drug. Known on the street as ice, blue, or crystal, this drug is more potent than amphetamines. This drug has no medicinal benefits. It is illegally produced in the United States and Mexico. Adverse effects include a decrease in cognitive and emotional functions, increased anxiety, and tooth decay.

Hallucinogens: A diverse group of drugs that alter a person's awareness of their surroundings, as well as their thoughts and feelings. Hallucinogens can be extracted from plants (mushrooms, peyote, and sativa) or can be man-made (LSD or PCP).

Ecstasy (MDMA): A synthetic drug that increases alertness, alters mood and perception, and emotional warmth.

GHB (Gamma Hydroxybutyrate): Commonly called the "date rape drug," it comes in liquid or powder form and has a salty taste when added to drinks. Effects include drowsiness, decreased anxiety, and hallucinations.

Depressants

These types of drugs are sometimes called "downers." Prescription antidepressants treat symptoms of depression and anxiety. These are known as tranquilizers or antipsychotics. All of these drugs carry a high risk for addiction.

Barbiturates/Benzodiazepines: Prescription drugs used to treat headaches, insomnia, and seizures. Used recreationally, these drugs can lead to addiction.

Opioids

Drugs originating from the seed pod of the opium poppy plant. Morphine is the purest form of this drug. These drugs bind to the body's opioid receptors and affect pain, pleasure, heart rate, sleep, and breathing.

Heroin: Made from morphine, heroin can be a white or brown powder or a black sticky substance known as "black tar heroin." Research has shown that prescription opioid drug misuse can lead to heroin use.

Prescription Opioids: Medications commonly used to treat pain. These include Vicodin, Norco, Percocet, and oxycontin. When used properly, these drugs are highly effective in treating pain. But due to their euphoric effects, they are often misused. Over the past 20 years, the United States has seen a surge in opioid abuse. The connection between these drugs and heroin use has been well documented. Patients misusing their pain medications may turn to street drugs (heroin and fentanyl) when their prescriptions run out.

Inhalants

Inhalants are gaseous drugs that sedate. These include nitrous oxide (laughing gas), poppers, and aerosols.

Recovery

All addictive substances cause discomfort in the user when they stop. Once medical intervention (detoxification) is completed, the patient can embark on the long and often difficult road to rehabilitation and recovery. Treatment courses vary and are dependent upon the user's ability to stay clean. Counseling with an addiction specialist, psychotherapist, or doctor are all steps in this process. Also, joining a support group that specializes in recovery from addiction is highly recommended.

Two of the more common support groups active worldwide are Alcoholics Anonymous (AA) and SMART. These programs are open to anyone who is seeking to stop their addiction and are FREE.

SMART Self-Management and Recovery Training: A self-empowering, non–12 step, mutual support program for addictive behaviors. This is a nonprofit organization that depends on grants and the support of others.

This program follows a 4-step progression to independence from addictive substances and behaviors. These steps are as follows:

- Building and maintaining motivation
- Coping with urges
- Managing thoughts, feelings, and behaviors
- Living a balanced life (www.smartrecovery.org, 2021)

Alcoholics Anonymous (AA): Another nonprofit organization, AA offers mutual support for those struggling with alcohol addiction. While they are not exclusive about the addiction type you have, most of those who attend these meetings are alcoholics. The only requirement for this program is having a desire to stop drinking.

This program is based on a 12-step process, outlined in their "Big Book." They also encourage some type of spirituality and promote sponsorship. A sponsor is someone who has gone through similar struggles and is there to assist the alcoholic with their own battles.

References

Colon-Rivera, H. (2020). "What Is addiction?" https://www.psychiatry.org/patients-families/addiction/whatisaddiction

Hardin, R. (2021). *SMART Recovery Handbook*, 3rd ed. Alcohol and Drug Abuse Self-Help Network. https://wwwsmartrecovery.org

Johnston, L., O'Malley, P., Miech, R., Bachman, J., & Schulenberg, J. (2015). Monitoring the Future National Survey Study. Study results on drug use: 1975–2015.

COMPLEMENTARY AND ALTERNATIVE MEDICINE, AGING, AND DEATH

CHAPTER 9

COMPLEMENTARY AND ALTERNATIVE MEDICINE

Integrative Medicine: An approach to health care putting the patient at the center of all dimensions of his or her health. Dimensions include physical, emotional, social, spiritual, intellectual, and environmental; treatment of the whole person.

Complementary Medicine: A non-mainstream practice that is used together with traditional Western medicine to treat and cure medical conditions.

Alternative Medicine: A non-mainstream medical practice that is used in place of traditional Western medicine.

Homeopathic Medicine (Natural): Embracing a natural approach to health. Using remedies produced according to the USFDA. No use of synthetic medications. Practitioners of this method believe in two tenets:

"Like cures like"—A disease can be cured by a substance that produces similar symptoms in healthy people.

"Law of minimum dose"—The lower the dose, the greater the effectiveness.

Naturopathy: Alternative medicine that treats disease without drugs through diet, exercise, and massage.

The National Center for Complementary and Integrative Health (NCCIH)

The NCCIH recognizes two subgroups in the complementary approaches:

Natural Products: Herbs, vitamins, minerals, and probiotics

Probiotics—Measures of potency are measured in colony-forming units (FUs). Live microorganisms and bacteria that are useful in managing digestion. Many of these products are similar to the natural bacteria that occur in the digestive tract. There is still much to be learned concerning the effectiveness of this additive.

Aromatherapy—The use of natural oils extracted from plants and flowers, applying the oil to the afflicted area or added to water and vaporized for inhalation. The scents can relieve stress, anxiety, insomnia, and many other conditions.

Mind and Body Practices: Massage therapy (most popular), Rolfing, yoga, Pilates, chiropractic and osteopathic manipulation, meditation, transcendental meditation, acupuncture, and relaxation techniques.

Also promotes hypnotherapy, tai chi, qigong, and movement therapies.

Feldenkrais Method—Exercise therapy that recognizes the connections between brain and body to improve body movement and psychological state

Alexander Technique—Learning to move "mindfully" through life

Trager Psychophysical Integration—Gentle, rhythmic rocking motion that brings the body and mind into sync, achieving a state of balance and integration

CHAPTER 10

AGING AND DEATH

GERONTOLOGY IS THE STUDY OF AGING. As we age, various functions of the body begin to slow down. The human body goes from generating tissues and organs to repairing and regenerating these physical components.

After age 30, the body slows its production of human growth hormone (HGH), a natural hormone that promotes tissue growth. The body eventually stops production altogether.

After age 40, the average American will lose 1% of their muscle mass, yearly. These processes go on and on, from generation to regeneration to degeneration; it's a fact of life. We can slow down and speed up this progression with modifiable lifestyle choices. Healthy eating and activity habits can slow the loss of muscle mass, but lifestyle choices like smoking or excessive drinking of alcohol will speed up the degeneration of the body's tissues, including the heart muscle.

The nonmodifiable aspects of our lives can't be changed. These include age, genetic history (having a predisposition to certain conditions thanks to our family tree), gender, and ethnicity.

So, what can you expect as you age?

Physical Changes

Heart: Heart rate slows, and arteries and veins become stiffer, causing the heart to work harder

Bones: Shrink in size and lose density, making them more fragile

Muscles: Lose strength and flexibility, causing a loss of coordination and trouble with balance

Gastrointestinal Tract: Chronic constipation or diarrhea. Usually due to low-fiber diet, lack of adequate hydration, and certain medications

Bladder: Urinary incontinence (trouble controlling urinary flow), many times due to menopause or prostate enlargement

Memory: Excluding the chronic conditions of dementia and Alzheimer's, memory loss is common as we age. Difficulty learning new concepts and problems remembering new words. Cognitive activity should be increased as we age. Taking classes, working puzzles, and reading are all types of these activities.

Eyes: Presbyopia; the lens in the eye becomes thin and rigid, disturbing the eye's ability to focus in the distance and up close.

Ears: Presbycusis; difficulty hearing

Teeth: Gums recede

Skin: Loss of elasticity, bruising more easily, decreased production of natural oils

Weight: As muscle mass decreases, body fat takes its place. Since muscle burns more fat than fat, this adds to one's weight.

Social Changes

As we get older, so do our friends and family, so loss of loved ones is not rare. Learning how to cope with these losses is a process that must be recognized.

Other changes include our ability to maintain our independence. Recognizing that we may not be capable of living alone, driving safely, or managing expenses well is very difficult to accept.

Social interaction begins to fall off in most seniors. Encouraging seniors in your life to get out of the house and engage in these types of interactions is very important.

Psychological Changes

Depression and Anxiety: Clinical depression and anxiety can go undiagnosed in seniors who shut themselves off to social interactions. Also, many seniors view mental illness as a weakness.

Dementia: Severe memory loss. A group of conditions characterized by two or more brain dysfunctions: forgetfulness, limited social skills and thinking ability, or loss of appropriate judgment, all interfering with daily functioning.

Alzheimer's Disease: A progressive disease that destroys memory. A degeneration of the neural pathways in the brain and the brain cells themselves. This affects cognitive, behavioral, mood, and psychological functions.

Legal End-of-Life Concerns

Living Will/Advanced Directive: A written statement of a person's wishes regarding their medical treatment. This is made to ensure that these wishes are carried out should the person become unable to communicate them. This must be witnessed by unrelated persons.

Legal Will: A legal document that expresses a person's (testator) wishes on how their property and assets are to be distributed upon their death. It also notes who will be designated the executor to manage these wishes.

Medical Care: Insurance and Medicare (a federal insurance plan available to those over 65 years of age).

Durable Power of Attorney: This gives someone you choose the power to act in your behalf if you become mentally incapable. There should be two of these documents: one that addresses health care decisions and one that covers financial decisions.

"Do Not Resuscitate" (DNR): At the patient's request, a medical order written by a doctor not to provide cardiopulmonary resuscitation (CPR) if the patient's heart stops beating.

Palliative Care: Patient care focusing on the patient's quality of life. This includes relief from symptoms and the stress of the illness. This is not hospice care. Palliative care is effected by a team of professionals, trained in caring for patients diagnosed with serious, chronic, or life-threatening illness. (www.getpalliativecare.org/ 2021)

Hospice Care: Provides compassionate care for people in the last phases of a terminal illness.

Hospice care focuses on providing for the patient in their last days or months of life, so that they can live as comfortably as possible during the time they have left. To qualify for hospice care, the doctors have determined that treatment is no longer working or the patient is ready to stop treatment. Patients may enter hospice care if they have a terminal illness or have been given 6 months or less to live. This can be done in the patient's home or in a care facility (American Cancer Society, 2019).

Death

Understanding Death: When there is a terminal diagnosis, both the patient and the family go through stages of coping. According to Dr. Elisabeth Kübler-Ross (*On Death and Dying,* 1969), recognizing these stages is the first step in coping with the inevitability of death and the eventual loss.

The five stages of dying/grief (or coming to terms with loss):

1. *Denial*
2. *Anger*
3. *Bargaining*
4. *Depression*
5. *Acceptance*

Death with Dignity Act (DWDA)

Passed in Oregon in 1997, the right to have physician-assisted suicide was made legal for those terminally ill patients diagnosed with less than 1 year to live. The number of states that have passed similar acts changes yearly.

Historically, death with dignity has been a hot topic in the United States. Dr. Jack Kevorkian, a pathologist in Michigan nicknamed "Dr. Death," offered his terminally ill patients physician-assisted suicide. While this service is still illegal in Michigan, Kevorkian provided this option to over 130 adults during the 1990s. In 1999, family members of several of his patients sued and took him to court, where he was convicted of manslaughter and served 8 years in prison. Kevorkian died of cancer in 2011.

Passive Euthanasia: Intentionally withholding life-sustaining treatment

Active Euthanasia: Life is terminated with the use of lethal drugs

Planning for the Inevitable: Organ donation

Taking care of your survivors; planning for after-death costs.

Burial or cremation?

References

Center to Advance Palliative Care. (2021). Retrieved June 3, 2021, from https://getpalliativecare.org/whatis/

Hospice Care. (2019, May 10). The American Cancer Society Medical and Editorial Content Team. Retrieved June 2, 2020, from https://www.cancer.org/treatment/endoflifecare/

Kübler-Ross, E. (1969). *On Death and Dying.* Macmillan.

"Palliative Care: Serious Illness: Get Palliative Care." Get Palliative Care Home Comments. Retrieved April 30, 2021, from http://www.getpalliativecare.org/

HUMAN SEXUALITY

CHAPTER 11

COMMUNICATION, RELATIONSHIPS, AND BEHAVIOR

Communication: A process by which information is exchanged between entities through a common system of symbols, signs, or behaviors

Relationships: The way in which two people communicate

Conflict Resolution: Discussion results in a remedy

    versus

Conflict Management: Discussion results in … "agreeing to disagree"

Sternberg's Triangular Theory of Love

Dr. Robert Sternberg created the triangular Theory of Love and identified three areas found in most human relationships. One or more of these areas can be found in most human relationships, depending on the type of love. He also identified seven types of love found in various relationships.

Table 11.1 defines the three components and identifies which components are found in that type of love. Note that "non-love" has none of the components and is not considered a type of love, but Sternberg does explain that non-love applies to strangers.

TABLE 11.1 Robert Sternberg's Triangular Theory and 7 Types of Love (Feurman, 2020)

Intimacy—meaningful communication
Passion—physical and emotional desires
Commitment—responsibility to another

	Intimacy	Passion	Commitment
Non-Love			
Liking	X		
Infatuation		X	
Empty			X
Companionate	X		X
Romantic	X	X	
Fatuous		X	X
Consummate	X	X	X

Hearing vs. Listening

Communication is the bedrock of a good relationship. There is a marked difference between hearing someone and listening to them. **Hearing** is the physiological act of perceiving sound. The act of hearing does not mean you are paying attention to what is being said. When you **hear someone talking**, you aren't always paying attention to what is being said. You know the person you are talking to is sharing with you, but you may be "somewhere else in your own head." **Listening to** someone during a conversation means you are engaged with the other person and are paying attention to what is being said. You are giving the words thoughtful consideration, and this improves communication.

Gender vs. Sex

Gender

Gender: One's feelings of being male or female

Sex: The anatomical, physiological assignment of one's maleness or femaleness

Gender Role: Set by society and based on one's biological assignment

Gender Identity: The gender with which one most closely identifies

How We Identify Ourselves

Cisgender: A person who identifies with their biological gender assignment

Nonbinary: Someone who does not identify as exclusively male or female. They may feel that their gender is a mixture of both male and female or that they have no gender at all.

Gender Nonconforming: Refers to those who do not adhere to society's rules about dress and activities for people that are based on their biological sex assignment

Androgynous: Possessing traditional traits of both genders

Transgender: Adjective used to describe those who identify with a gender identity other than their assigned gender at birth

One who pursues gender reassignment surgery is described as trans, BUT the labeling is mostly inaccurate. Sexual characteristics are changed through surgery and hormone therapy.

Sexual Relationships

Dr. Alfred Kinsey was one of the most recognized scientists in the area of human sexuality. The Kinsey reports began in 1948. The following represent terms related to sexual relationships:

Sexual Orientation: Term to describe an individual's specific experience with physical, romantic and/or emotional attraction to others.

Heterosexual: Adjective typically used to describe those attracted to the opposite sex. This word is still used but the definition is vague.

Homosexual (Gay): Adjective used to describe members of the LGBTQIA+ community. Typically used to describe those attracted to the same sex.

Bisexual (Pansexual): Adjective used to describe people who experience physical, romantic and/or emotional attraction to multiple orientations. Most do not have equal preference for who they are attracted to.

Asexual: Adjective used to describe people who experience little to no sexual attraction to others regardless of gender or sexual orientation. An umbrella term for the asexuality spectrum that includes other orientations related to emotional and romantic attraction.

Sexual Behaviors

Erogenous Zones—anywhere on the body that has a heightened sensitivity that elicits a sexual response

Masturbation—sexual self-pleasuring

Oral Sex—cunnilingus, or the oral stimulation of the female genitalia; fellatio, or the oral stimulation of the male genitalia

Sodomy—sexual intercourse involving anal or oral sex. This practice is codified in many state laws as an unnatural act and may be deemed as illegal.

Vaginal Intercourse—penile penetration of the vagina

Anal Intercourse—penile penetration of the anus into the rectum

Sexual Fantasies—healthy sexual expression of sexual desires and kinks

Paraphilias:

Frequent, intense, sexually arousing fantasies or behaviors that involve inanimate objects, children of nonconsenting adults, or suffering or humiliation of oneself or a partner.

Noncoercive—solo activities or activities that involve consenting adults.

Coercive—paraphilic disorder. These impulses become difficult to control. These may include (but are not limited to) voyeurism, frotteurism, bestiality, or pedophilia. The APA refuses to classify coercive pedophilia in the DSM-V, stating that these behaviors are not psychiatric behaviors and instead, when involving victims, should be considered criminal activity.

Intimate, Passionate, Committed Relationships

- *Cohabitation*—sharing bed and board
- *Common law marriage*—a couple is legally considered married without formally registering civilly. The amount of time they have lived together varies from state to state.
- *Domestic partnership and civil union*—legally recognized union of two individuals
- *Marriage*—a personal relationship arising out of a civil contract between two people who are capable of making the contract, are unmarried, over 18 years of age, and not otherwise disqualified. They are both capable of consenting to and consummating marriage.
- *Palimony*—alimony for unmarried cohabiting couples
- *Divorce*—legal dissolution of a marriage

Reference

Feurman, M. (2020). Sternberg's Triangular Theory and 7 Types of Love. https://www.verywellmind.com/types-of-love-we-experience-2303200

CHAPTER 12

REPRODUCTIVE ANATOMY
AND SEXUAL PHYSIOLOGY

Female Sexual Anatomy

The three main functions of the exterior sexual anatomy:

- Enable sperm to enter the body

- Protect internal organs

- Provide sexual pleasure

Exterior Structures

- Vulva (mons pubis)—rounded mass of fatty tissue that covers the pubic bone. During puberty it becomes covered in hair. Its sebaceous glands release substances (pheromones) involved in sexual attraction.

- Labia majora ("large lips")—fleshy folds of tissue that enclose and protect the external genital organs. These are homologous to the scrotum in males.

- Labia minora ("small lips")—these lie just inside the labia majora and surround the openings to the vagina and urethra.

- Clitoris—located between the upper end of the labia majora and the upper part of the labia minora, it is a small "button" that plays a major role in female sexual excitement. Homologous to the penis.

- Clitoral hood—female foreskin

- Perineum—an imaginary line (tissue) between the vagina and the anus. Sometimes this is surgically cut to allow for childbirth.

- Bartholin's glands—located beside the vaginal opening, they secrete a thick fluid that supplies lubrication during sexual excitement.

- Hymen—a thin, temporary membrane located at the opening to the vagina. This tissue has been linked to virginity in many cultures.

Interior Structures

- Urethral opening—entry to the urethra

- Urethra—vessel that transports urine from the bladder

- Urinary bladder—holds urine

- Vagina—tubelike, muscular, elastic organ about 4 to 5 inches long. Organ of sexual intercourse; passage for childbirth and menses as it leaves the body.

- Cervix—entry to the uterus from the vagina

- Uterus—organ that sustains life during pregnancy; develops menstrual product and contracts during labor.

- Fallopian tubes (2)—passageways for an egg from ovaries to the uterus. Primary site for fertilization.

- Fimbriae (2 sets)—small, fingerlike structures that guide the egg from the ovary into the fallopian tube during ovulation

- Ovaries (2)—the size of a walnut, these two structures produce the female hormones (estrogen and progesterone) and produce and release eggs

   o *Eggs cells (oocytes) are contained inside follicles until ovulation. On average, women are born with approximately 300 oocytes. When she has released her last egg, the woman is no longer fertile. This is called menopause.*

- Anus

- Rectum

Male Sexual Anatomy

Exterior

- Scrotum—Homologous to the labia majora in women, this sac of skin hangs below the penis and holds the testicles and the epididymis. It is responsible for maintaining the temperature of the testicles at 5 to 6 degrees below body temperature. If temperature within the scrotum is too high or too low, it can cause damage to the developing sperm.

   o *The cremaster muscle is responsible for pulling the scrotum closer to the body or releasing it away from the body in order to maintain this temperature.*

- Testicles (2)—Homologous to the ovaries, they produce sperm and the male sex hormone, testosterone. The process of sperm production is called spermatogenesis.

- Epididymides (2)—located at the top of each testicle, these structures house mature sperm until ejaculation. A small amount of semen is produced within the epididymis for sperm nourishment.

Interior

- Vas deferens (2)—long, narrow tubes that transport the ejaculate. These eventually merge with the urethra at the seminal vesicles.

- Seminal vesicles (2)—small organs that produce semen, responsible for the majority of the fluid during ejaculation, 60%. This fluid consists mostly of a fructose-rich substance providing energy for the sperm and a neutralizing agent necessary for cleansing the male urethra and the vagina.

- Ejaculatory ducts (2)—found at the base of the seminal vesicles, these are the exit ways for semen into the vas deferens.

- Prostate gland—this gland produces fluid that assists in sperm mobility. During ejaculation, the gland closes off the urethra, keeping urine out of the ejaculate. Making up approximately 30% of the semen, this fluid also helps protect the sperm as they make their way to the egg. It is the size of a walnut and is sensitive to pressure, which may create sexual pleasure.

- Urinary bladder—site of urine storage

- Urethra—a tube that carries ejaculate and urine out of the body

- Cowper's gland—this gland holds pre-ejaculate. During ejaculation, this gland collects the last 5% of the ejaculate and holds it until the next ejaculation. This fluid is released prior to ejaculation and is called pre-ejaculate. Released during the plateau stage of the sexual response, it can cause pregnancy.

- Penis—made up of three spongy layers called cavernosum, its average size is 5 to 7 inches when erect. When sexual excitement occurs, the cavernosum become engorged with blood (vasocongestion), making the penis hard.

- Foreskin—thin, protective flap of skin covering the glans. Some men have this removed at birth (circumcision).

- Frenulum—the area where the foreskin meets the underside of the penis. It looks like a small *V* just below the glans. Possessing many nerve endings, this is a very sensitive area.

- Glans penis—the "head" of the penis

- Anus

- Rectum

Sexual Development

Female: Puberty occurs between the ages of 8 to 13 with menarche (first menstruation) and lasts 3 to 4 years. Development includes breast growth, erratic emotions, acne, body odor, and mood swings. During this stage in life, the female will begin the capacity to reproduce and will take on adult characteristics. These changes are regulated by hormones produced in the pituitary gland (LH and FSH). These hormones stimulate the production of progesterone and estrogen by the ovaries.

Women will go through three distinctive phases of reproductive function:
- Menarche—first menstruation
- Menstruation—the monthly cycle of endometrial buildup and release of an egg

- *Perimenopause—the first stage of menopause. This is a transition stage to menopause. It can begin as early as age 40 and ends with menopause. Symptoms include hot flashes, sleep disturbances, mood changes, vaginal dryness, and headaches.*

- Menopause—the woman has released all of her eggs and is no longer fertile.

    - *Postmenopause—no menstrual cycle for a minimum of 12 months*

Worldwide cultural practices associated with female sexual development (none of the following have any medical significance):

1. Female Genital Mutilation (FGM)
2. Clitoridectomy—removal of clitoral hood and all or part of the clitoris
3. Excision—removal of clitoris and labia minora
4. Infibulation—narrowing of the vaginal opening by surgically cutting and restitching the labia majora

These practices are most common in North Africa (from Gambia on the west coast to Ethiopia on the east), Iraq, Yemen, Southeast Asia, and the Middle East. It is illegal to perform these procedures on minor females in the United States.

Male: Puberty occurs between ages 10 to 15 and lasts for 3 to 4 years before sexual maturity is reached. Physiological and psychological changes include erratic emotions, facial hair, acne, stunted or slow growth, voice changes, mood swings, unwanted erections, and body odor, and some may develop small breasts that eventually go away within a year.

Worldwide cultural rituals to manhood:

1. Circumcision—removal of the foreskin, usually occurring at birth. In the Jewish faith, this procedure is done 8 days after birth. It becomes more difficult, complicated, and riskier in older children and men. Infant circumcision takes about 10 minutes, while in adults it can take up to an hour.
2. Naked bull jumping—in Ethiopia, boys must be able to run across a row of bulls several times without falling before they can be a father. If a boy fathers a child before completing this ritual, he must kill the newborn or the mother must leave the child in the wilderness until the boy can successfully complete the ritual.
3. Sambia tribe clubhouse—at age 7, boys are removed from their mother's company and forced to live with a group of tribal males. They are given regular nosebleeds and must consume semen regularly (considered essential to encouraging masculine growth and development). Multiple stages must be achieved before reaching manhood.
4. Zulu "man camp"—teens are taken into the wilderness where they learn how to be men. The ceremony of circumcision includes being covered in white dust and being circumcised by a drunken witch doctor. If they survive, they live for another month in naked seclusion.

There are multiple rituals and ceremonies recognizing manhood supported by cultures worldwide. Above are just a few examples.

Human Sexual Response

Doctors William Masters and Virginia Johnson conducted multiple human studies surrounding the human sexual response and found that men and women go through four distinct stages, from sexual excitement through orgasm. These stages are as follows:

Excitement—initial response to sexual stimulation

Plateau—anatomical structures prepare for orgasm; penis becomes fully erect, vagina forms seminal pool

Orgasm—muscular contractions in and around the genitalia; release of seminal fluids

Resolution—body returns to pre-excited state (Masters & Johnson, 1966).

Disorders of the Reproductive System

Female Sexual Dysfunction

Persistent, recurring problems with sexual response, desire, function, or pain. These problems can occur for many different reasons, most commonly when hormones are in flux, after pregnancy, or during menopause. Major illnesses can also contribute to these problems, as well as STIs. Also, many drug therapies (antidepressants, high blood pressure medicines, antihistamines, and chemotherapy) can decrease sexual desire.

Amenorrhea: The absence of menstruation. Diagnosed as a disorder if one misses three or more periods in a row.

Premenstrual Syndrome (PMS): A group of symptoms that occur monthly prior to the onset of menstruation. Symptoms include mood swings, tender breasts, fatigue, abdominal cramping, irritability, depression, food cravings.

Premenstrual Dysphoric Disorder (PMDD): A more severe form of PMS.

Dyspareunia: Painful intercourse; the vaginal lining becomes thinner, less elastic, and may not lubricate. Could also be due to sores on the inner walls of the vagina.

Vaginismus: Muscle spasms within the vagina during or prior to penetration, causing the vagina to tighten.

Endometriosis: When the tissue that lines the interior of the uterus (endometrium) migrates outside of the uterus and attaches to the outer walls of the ovaries, fallopian tubes, intestines, and other organs in the pelvic region.

Polycystic Ovarian Syndrome (PCOS): The growth of cysts in the ovaries, interfering with ovulation.

Male Sexual Dysfunction

Causes may include inherited disorders, hormonal imbalance, dilated veins around the testicles, or a blockage of the vas deferens. Some drugs and specific medical conditions can also interrupt sexual function.

Premature Ejaculation: Ejaculation before the completion of the sex act. One in three males will experience this in their lifetime.

Retrograde Ejaculation: Ejaculate goes into the bladder instead of exiting the penis.

Erectile Dysfunction (Impotence): The inability to get and/or keep an erection firm enough for sex.

Peyronie's Disease: Inadequate blood flow to one of the corpus cavernosum, or scarring inside these chambers. This causes a painful bend of the penis during an erection.

Hypogonadism: The testicles do not produce adequate amounts of testosterone or sperm. This interferes with the male's ability to reproduce.

Epididymal Hypertension: Pain/aching of the testicles after vasocongestion without ejaculation.

Reference

Masters, W., & Johnson, V. (1966). Retrieved from https://www.goodtherapy.org/famous-psychologists/william-masters.html

CHAPTER 13

REPRODUCTION

Reproduction

Fertilization (Conception): The union of the egg and sperm, most commonly occurring in the fallopian tube following intercourse. Within hours of fertilization, the **zygote** is formed, and for approximately 5 days, this cluster of cells moves through the fallopian tube to the uterus, where it develops into a **blastocyst**. The blastocyst implants into the uterus, where the inner layers will become the **embryo,** and the outer layers will become the **placenta**. For the next 8 weeks, the embryo begins to grow, beginning with the development of the brain and the central nervous system. At the eighth week, the embryo become a **fetus**. It is attached to the placenta via the **umbilical cord** in order to receive nutrients from the mother; the fetus is surrounded by the **amniotic sac**, which is full of amniotic fluid. This fluid contains important DNA information about the fetus and protects the fetus from trauma.

Infertility

Infertility is the inability to get pregnant, despite you and your partner having frequent, unprotected sex for at least 1 year.

Causes:

Female—ovulation problems, age, scar tissue buildup, inhospitable uterus, and some chronic diseases

Male—low sperm count, low testosterone, misshapen or immobile sperm, scar tissue buildup, and the inability to ejaculate

Behaviors that may interfere with fertility include tobacco or cannabis smoking, alcohol and other drug use, being overweight or underweight, and STIs. In women, excessive exercise and inadequate levels of body fat. In men, wearing tight underwear/pants and frequent hot tub use.

Treatments and Options for Infertility:

- Fertility drugs—Mostly for women, these drugs trigger the release of multiple eggs at one ovulation. Treatment is continued for up to 6 months. Males who are experiencing low testosterone may receive testosterone injections or be prescribed the testosterone patch.

- Intrauterine insemination (IUI)—A concentrated amount of sperm is artificially introduced to the female sexual anatomy with hopes of meeting with an awaiting egg.

- Donor egg—The male's sperm are placed in his partner's uterus, where a donated egg is waiting to be fertilized.

- In vitro fertilization (IVF)—Both sperm and egg are handled and introduced in the laboratory setting, forming an embryo that is then introduced into the uterus.

- Gamete intrafallopian transfer (GIFT)—Eggs are collected from the female and placed in the fallopian tube. The couple is then encouraged to engage in intercourse immediately, promoting natural fertilization. The result becomes a zygote, which makes its way to the uterus for natural implantation.

- Zygote intrafallopian transfer (ZIFT)—The egg and sperm are collected and introduced in the lab; then, the resulting zygotes are artificially introduced into the fallopian tube. From there, the zygote makes its way to the uterus where it implants.

- Surrogacy—A host uterus (woman) is hired for the 9 months of pregnancy. She carries another couple's biological fetus and gives it to that couple after childbirth. The contract between the couple and the host must be clear and legally binding. All costs for this pregnancy are covered by the couple.

- Adoption—An infertile couple seeks out a woman who has given birth and cannot keep her baby. This is best done through a third party to ensure that all legal issues are covered.

  Costs for all of these procedures may vary dependent upon the third party's involvement.

Pregnancy

Prenatal Care: Regular doctors' visits ensuring that the mother is healthy and consuming enough calories to maintain a healthy pregnancy. Tests may be performed prior to birth the ensure the health of the developing fetus.

Tests:

- Ultrasound
- Amniocentesis
- Alpha-fetoprotein blood test
- Chorionic villus sampling

Trimesters: Three 13-week divisions of a healthy pregnancy

Trimester 1—Fertilization to beginnings of fetal development. This is the foundation for the entire pregnancy. All major organs begin to develop.

Trimester 2—Fetal growth, continuation of organ development, and forming and development of the musculoskeletal system. The fetus will grow to approximately 15 in. long and will weigh up to 2 lbs. This will last until the 26th week.

Trimester 3—The majority of fetal growth will happen during this stage, culminating with the birth. Also part of this phase is the delivery of the placenta. After the umbilical cord is cut, the woman's contractions should continue until her body expels the placenta.

Multiple births (twins, triplets, sometimes called multiples)—This may occur if there was more than one egg present during fertilization or one or more of the eggs split prior to implantation. Most common in women on fertility drugs, there are two types of multiples.

Identical: come from the same egg that has split

Fraternal: occurs when more than one egg is fertilized by separate sperm

Birthing Complications

Miscarriage: Loss of a pregnancy that usually occurs before the third month. Most times the cause is not known, and some women don't even know that they were pregnant.

Preeclampsia: Characterized by high blood pressure, protein in the urine, and edema showing up after the 20th week; 5% to 10% percent of pregnancies will involve preeclampsia. If not recognized and treated, it can progress to eclampsia, which may put the pregnancy at risk, as well as the mother's life. Risk factors for preeclampsia include pregnancy with multiple babies, being older than 35, or being in your early teens, first pregnancy, obesity, high blood pressure, or diabetes.

Eclampsia: A severe complication of untreated preeclampsia. Symptoms include high blood pressure, seizures, or unexplained coma during the last months of pregnancy. Usually occurs after the 20th month and is life threatening.

Ectopic Pregnancy: When a fertilized egg attaches itself outside of the uterus. Occurs in one of every 50 pregnancies. Treatment depends on the location of the implanted blastocyte.

Placenta Previa: Occurs in the last months of pregnancy. The placenta drops down and covers or partially covers the cervix, blocking the exit of the fetus. Diagnosis and treatment depend on how much of the cervix is covered.

Breech Birth: The baby has not moved into the headfirst position in preparation for birth. Positions include the following:

- Footling breech—one foot or both present first
- Frank breech—bottom first
- Complete breech—bottom first with legs crossed

If this occurs, doctors will first try the external cephalic version of delivery, which requires doctors to manually turn the baby into the headfirst position. This usually occurs at 37 weeks.

Birthing Options

Prior to childbirth, there are several options a woman has for giving birth.

- Unassisted childbirth (natural)—no medical interventions, including pain medications. About 2% will choose to deliver their baby at home. This is usually attended by a midwife.
- Lamaze technique—pre-birth classes focus on breathing and partner assistance
- Bradley method—focus on breathing and partner support
- Water birth—happens in a large tub about the size of a hot tub

All of these are vaginal births, which have many more positives than a surgical removal of the baby. Positive side effects of vaginal births include:

- Infants with fewer respiratory problems
- Mom recovers more quickly
- Lower rates of infection and shorter hospital stays

Birthing Procedures Done in the Hospital

Vacuum Extraction: If the fetus is not leaving the uterus but has moved into the proper headfirst position, the doctor may opt to help it along using this procedure. A soft cup is attached to the fetus's head and a handheld pump is used to create suction to remove it. While there is less fetal distress than a C-section, there are risks of scalp injuries, trauma, or bleeding of the head.

Forceps Delivery: A curved instrument with clamps is used to facilitate the progress of the fetus in the birth canal.

Cesarean Section (C-section): Surgical removal of the fetus through the abdomen. One-third of births in the United States are done by C-section. Experts say this number should be around 15%, but higher rates are due to elective C-sections and physician overuse.

Labor

Every woman's labor is unique and different. There is no way to accurately predict exactly when a woman will go into labor.

Braxton-Hicks Contractions: False labor. Contractions are milder than true labor. The pregnant woman may experience a burst of energy and an increased urge for a bowel movement.

Lightening: The fetal head drops down into the pelvis. This may occur 2 weeks prior to delivery. This may cause an increased urge to urinate.

There are three stages of labor during childbirth.

Stage 1—Early Labor and Active Labor

This is the longest stage of labor.

Early: Beginning of contractions and cervical dilation. The amniotic sac ruptures, releasing the amniotic fluid (water breaking). The **mucus plug** (a thick mass that covers the cervix during pregnancy) must be dispelled before childbirth can occur and may be dispelled during this stage. Not time for the hospital yet.

Active: Contractions are stronger and closer in time, with a cervical dilation of about 10 centimeters. NOW is the time to go to the hospital. This may last 8 hours or longer. The last part of active labor is called transition.

Stage 2—Birth of the Baby

The woman is instructed to push as the baby leaves the uterus through the cervix and into the birth canal (vagina). The baby's head appears (crowning). Once head is out, the rest of the baby follows. At this time, the doctor or midwife will remove the mucus from the baby's airway and cut the umbilical cord.

Stage 3—Delivery of the Placenta

This typically takes from 5 to 30 minutes following the delivery of the baby. The doctor will check the placenta and clear any remaining remnants from the uterus. They will also repair the perineum if there was any tearing.

When do doctors induce?

- One week after due date
- "Water" breaks and labor doesn't begin
- Placenta stops functioning
- Mother develops preeclampsia
- Mother has an illness that threatens her health
- Mother has a history of stillbirths

Sudden Infant Death Syndrome (SIDS): Sudden, unexplained death of an infant under the age of 1 year. Nearly always associated with sleep. Infants affected with this are otherwise healthy. Doctors hypothesize that something happens in the baby's brain affecting breathing. Infants with low birth weight or that are premature are most at risk due to the underdevelopment of the brain and lungs.

Making sure that the baby sleeps unencumbered by blankets, pillows, stuffed animals, and family pets are all important in avoiding breathing problems.

Breastfeeding: Generally recommended for the first 12 months of life, according to the American Academy of Pediatrics (AAP). Colostrum is the first form of milk produced by the mammary glands of mammals immediately following delivery of a newborn. Mothers will produce colostrum for 3 to 4 days before "mature milk" comes in. Colostrum is a nutrient-rich fluid, loaded with immune, growth, and tissue repair factors. It helps with the development of immunity in newborns. It also helps prevent jaundice and low blood sugar and helps build a strong immune system in the newborn.

Positives of breastfeeding: superior nutrition, increased resistance to infection, decreased risk of allergies and lactose intolerance; breast milk is sterile, reduced risk of thrush

Negatives of breastfeeding: inconvenient; nursing in public can be stressful; pain or discomfort

Baby Blues: The emotional state that follows childbirth. This includes tearfulness, worry, fatigue, self-doubt, and unhappiness; it should go away within 2 weeks of giving birth.

Postpartum Mood Disorder (PPD)

About 15% of new mothers will experience PPD, sometimes referred to as perinatal disease. Symptoms may occur a few days after delivery or as late as 1 year after giving birth. Symptoms will vary and can be mild to severe. They usually last for about 2 weeks. Symptoms include fatigue, feelings of being overwhelmed, sadness, hopelessness, and trouble eating or sleeping. There may also be feelings of guilt or worthlessness, withdrawing from family members, lack of interest in the baby, and thoughts of hurting oneself or the baby (National Institute of Mental Health).

Subgroups:

- Postpartum Anxiety (PPA)—Can include panic attacks

- Postpartum obsessive-compulsive disorder (PPOCD)—This manifests as an over-preoccupation with the baby. Keeping the baby safe or even fear of being alone with the baby become all encompassing.

- Postpartum post-traumatic stress (PPPTSD)—Occurs in women who experience real or perceived trauma directly following childbirth.

Reference

U.S. Department of Health and Human Services. (n.d.). *Perinatal Depression*. National Institute of Mental Health. Retrieved June 3, 2021, from https://www.nimh.nih.gov/health/publications/perinatal-depression/#pub5

FAMILY PLANNING
AND BIRTH CONTROL

Birth Control

Considering safety and what works for you, make your choices based on the following:

- Use compatibility and convenience
- STI protection
- Reversibility
- Typical use effectiveness
- Continuation rate
- Contraceptive failure rate

Preventing Pregnancy

Options fall into four categories: natural, barrier, hormonal (chemical), surgical

1. **Natural**
   a. <u>Non-procreative abstinence</u>—100% effective; not engaging in vaginal intercourse
   b. <u>Withdrawal</u>—78% effective; coitus interruptus, the withdrawing of the penis from the vagina before ejaculation
   c. <u>Family awareness methods (FAM)</u>—76% to 88% effective, this charts the woman's ovulation. This method can also be used to plan for pregnancy.
   d. <u>FAM 1- Calendar method</u>—keeping track of the most fertile point of a woman's cycle. This is done by counting the number of days between the beginning and end of bleeding and then determining ovulation (when the egg is present in the fallopian tube).
   e. <u>FAM 2- Temperature method</u>—basal body temperature (BBT); checking temperature daily to notice an increase of 0.8 degrees over 2 days. This may indicate ovulation.

f. <u>FAM 3—Vaginal mucus method (Billings method)</u>—daily checking of the consistency of vaginal mucus, which normally is sticky and cloudy. At ovulation, it takes on the consistency of an uncooked egg white.

g. <u>Lactation amenorrhea</u>—98% effective because while breastfeeding the woman does not ovulate. This is only effective for up to 12 weeks after delivery.

2. **Barrier**
   a. <u>Male condoms</u>—85% effective; latex or other substance sheath covering the erect penis; designed to collect ejaculate so it does not enter the female reproductive system

   b. <u>Female condoms</u>—79% effective; polyurethane sheath inserted into the vagina with a purpose similar to the male condom

   c. <u>Contraceptive sponge</u>—76% to 86% effective; self-inserted 24 hours or less prior to intercourse. This sponge should cover the cervix. Moisten and squeeze until sudsy. The suds contain spermicide. One-time use only.

   d. <u>Cervical cap</u>—71% to 86% effective; sailor's cap–shaped cover for the cervix. Can be left in place for 2 days. Reusable.

   e. <u>Diaphragm</u>—88% effective; small and saucer-shaped, it is inserted into the vagina to cover the cervix. Must be fitted by a doctor. Remove after sex act. Reusable.

   f. <u>Intrauterine device (IUD)</u>—99% effective; inserted into the uterus by a doctor. Interferes with sperm mobility and secretes hormones or copper ions. Five brands to choose from in the United States:
      o *Para-Gard: uses copper ions (no hormones) to interfere with sperm. Travels to find the egg; lasts 10 years.*
      o *Mirena: uses progestin to slow progression of sperm; lasts 6 years*
      o *Kyleena: hormonal; lasts 5 years*
      o *Liletta: hormonal; lasts 4 years*
      o *Skyla: hormonal; lasts 3 years*

3. **Hormonal (Chemical)**
   a. <u>Oral birth control (OC)</u>—91% effective; birth control pills
      o *Combination pills: contain both estrogen and progestin*
      o *Mini-pills: progestin only*
      o *Must be taken every day at the same time*

   b. <u>The Patch</u>—91% effective; a transdermal application left in place for one week; dispenses estrogen and progestin

   c. <u>Vaginal contraceptive ring</u>—91% effective; the NuvaRing has estrogen and progestin; it is left in place and changed once a month

d. <u>Implant (Nexplanon)</u>—99% effective; one matchstick-size rod inserted under the skin on the inside of the left upper arm. This will secrete progestin for up to 4 years.

e. <u>Injection (Depo-Provera)</u>—94% effective; lasts for 3 months; a more powerful progestin is used for this type of BC

4. **Chemical**

a. <u>Spermicide</u>—Spermicidal substance that is 71% effective when used alone. Comes in gel, cream, or foam. This should be used with a barrier birth control method.

5. **Surgical**

Both methods have a 99% effectiveness rate.

Invasive procedures used to block eggs or sperm from leaving the body.

a. *Female*: <u>Tubal ligation</u>—fallopian tubes are cut and stapled or burned, blocking the egg's route to the uterus. This creates scar tissue, damaging the tubes. It is not easily reversed.

b. *Male:* <u>Vasectomy</u>—vas deferens is cut and tied or stapled, blocking the sperms' pathway out of the body. This is reversible.

Emergency Contraception

None of these measures should be used as primary birth control, as the substances used are tough on the body. The following methods stop ovulation but do not stop pregnancy. These are NOT abortion pills.

Plan B: Called "next chance," "my way," "one step," etc., these can all be gotten without a prescription and will work up to 5 days following unprotected sex, BUT they do lose some of their effectiveness over time.

<u>Ella</u>—the hormone ulipristal; it blocks the hormones needed for conception. Good for 5 days after unprotected sex and DOES NOT lose effectiveness over the 5 days. Requires a prescription.

<u>ParaGard IUD</u>—the insertion of this IUD blocks conception while secreting progesterone to stop ovulation. It can be left in place for 10 years.

Unwanted Pregnancy

ABORTION: In 1973, the court case of *Roe v. Wade* made it legal in the United States to have an abortion (the purposeful termination of a pregnancy) up to the third month of pregnancy. Today, abortion laws vary from state to state. Someone seeking an abortion should check the laws in their state to see how late in pregnancy abortions are allowed (Planned Parenthood, 2021).

In 2017, 18% of pregnancies (excluding miscarriages) ended in abortion, down 7% from 2014. These numbers continue to decline.

While abortion rates have declined in the United States, it is still a very controversial subject. The two sides of this debate, pro-life and pro-choice, continue to fight for and against these rights. Twenty states in the United States are considered to be "anti-abortion right states," and legislation concerning these rights appears on almost every ballot during election years.

Unsafe abortions are those performed by unqualified persons and in unsafe environments without follow-up care. Worldwide, 45% of all abortions are unsafe. Almost all of these are carried out in developing countries (Guttmacher Institute, 2021).

There are two drug therapies used to cause chemical abortion. These medications should only be used once pregnancy is confirmed and is unwanted. These drugs are as follows:

RU 486: "Abortion pill"; a two-step process, usually referred to as a <u>medication abortion</u>.

There are two drugs used with this method:

<u>Mifepristone</u>—can be taken within 4 weeks of unprotected sex and up to 11 weeks. It acts on the uterus by not allowing the endometrium to build up and by blocking the hormone needed for pregnancy.

<u>Misoprostol</u>—The second pill is taken 6 to 72 hours later. This causes severe uterine contractions, emptying the uterus of any remaining contents. It can also cause severe bleeding.

Symptoms: Cramping, pain, heavy bleeding, and large clots from the vagina. Also, headaches, nausea, vomiting, chills, and diarrhea. Light bleeding may continue up to 4 weeks following treatment.

Surgical Abortion: Use of invasive measures to end a pregnancy.

<u>Manual vacuum aspiration</u>: Can be performed up to 12 weeks following unprotected sex if a pregnancy occurs; a syringe is inserted into the uterus and a vacuum removes the contents.

<u>Dilation and evacuation (D & E)</u>: After the first month and up to the 24th week, this type of abortion removes all contents from the uterus using a tool to scrape the interior.

<u>Late-term abortion (dilation and extraction or D&X)</u>: Third-trimester (24 weeks) abortions are illegal in 40 states and the District of Columbia and may only be performed if the mother's life is at risk. These are sometimes referred to as "partial birth abortions."

References

Guttmacher Institute. (2021). Retrieved on June 4, 2021, from https://www.guttmacher.org/fact-sheet/induced-abortion-unitedstates#

Planned Parenthood. (2021). https://www.plannedparenthoodaction.org/issues/abortion/roe-v-wade 2021

DISEASE

CHAPTER 15

COMMUNICABLE DISEASE

Human Immune System

The human immune system is made up of white blood cells that are produced and stored in the lymphatic system. The immune system is called into action when antigens (any agent that sparks an immune response) are recognized.

There are numerous types of cells in the immune system, and each has a specific job to do. The following are just three of these cells.

Macrophages: patrol for pathogens and remove dead cells

Leukocytes: T-cells destroy damaged and mutated cells

B-cells: produce antibodies to fight specific invading cells

Pus: a thick, greenish-yellow liquid produced by infected tissue that indicates infection. Made up of white blood cells, bacteria, tissue debris, and serum.

Chain of Infection

Pathogen

Reservoir

Portal of exit

Mode of transmission

Portal of entry

Infectious Agents

- **Infection:** The effect of foreign organisms on the body

  The most common infectious diseases found in the United States include the common cold, flu, strep throat, urinary tract infections (UTIs), pneumonia, and STIs.

- **Vectors:** Disease-carrying agents include insects, animals, people, water, and food.

- **Pathogens:** Germs. Groups of pathogens include:

- *Bacteria*—single-celled agents. Some require a host and some do not. Infections are treated with antibiotics.
  Examples: methicillin-resistant *Staphylococcus aureus* (MRSA), meningitis, TB, pink eye

- *Virus*—smallest of the pathogens. Must have a host to survive. There are no cures for viral infections, but some viral infections can be avoided by getting vaccinated.
  Examples: common cold, flu, meningitis, chicken pox

- *Fungi, mold, and yeast*—organisms that absorb their food from organic matter. These can be cured with specific medications, both topical and oral.
  Examples: athlete's foot, ringworm, yeast infections

- *Protozoa*—single-celled organisms that can live both inside and outside the body. Treated with oral medications.
  Examples: meningitis, amebic dysentery, malaria

- *Parasites and worms*—multi-celled organisms that live off the host doing damage and causing disease. These creatures do not survive long without a host.
  Examples: ticks, fleas, bedbugs, head and body lice, worms (roundworms, tapeworms, flukes)

Sexually Transmitted Infections (STIs, Previously Called STDs)

- 1 in 4 college students today has some form of STI.
- The only way to be 100% protected from these infections is to abstain from sexual contact.
- 80% of individuals with an STI experience no noticeable symptoms.

General signs of STIs include sores/blisters, rash, penile or vaginal discharge, painful urination, abdominal pain, or none at all (Kaufman, 2020).

Types of STIs

1. Human papilloma virus (HPV), condyloma (genital warts)—An infection that occurs when you come in contact with the infectious wart.

   HPV most commonly appears in

   Females: vulva, labia, vaginal walls, cervix

   Males: glans penis, penis, scrotum

   There is a vaccine for this virus.

2. Herpes simplex virus types 1 and 2 (HSV 1 & 2)—Viral disease transmitted through contact with infectious sores. There is no cure and no vaccine for herpes.

   Type 1: the sores appear on the lips or around the mouth

   Type 2: the sores appear around the genitals or inside the labia and vagina

   Treatment includes oral meds such as acyclovir and mega-dosing with the amino acid lysine, ice directly on the site of the developing sore, and topical medications.

3. Human immunodeficiency virus (HIV)—There is no cure and no vaccine for this virus. The virus mimics and hides inside healthy cells. With proper treatment, this disease can be kept at a manageable state. If it does progress, the diagnosis can become acquired immunodeficiency syndrome (AIDS). Most common symptoms for AIDS include Kaposi's sarcoma (cancer), pneumocystis carinii, pneumonia (PCP), dementia, and wasting syndrome. These are all "opportunistic infections," which generally do not affect those with healthy immune systems.

4. Chlamydia—A bacterial infection spread through sexual contact with infected fluids, primarily vaginal secretions and semen. Symptoms appear approximately 7 days following contact and include foul-smelling discharge that is greenish-yellow, burning pain during urination, and extreme itchiness around the genitals. This is easily treated with antibiotics. If not treated, it can lead to pelvic inflammatory disease (PID).

5. Gonorrhea—A bacterial infection that can be transmitted through contact with infected secretions or contact with a gonococcal sore. After infection, it can take up to 6 months before symptoms appear. Initial symptoms include burning urination, raised sore on area of contact with infected fluids, and discharge from urethra or vagina. Treatment includes antibiotics. Without treatment, PID can occur.

6. Syphilis—These bacteria are called spirochetes and are much more difficult to eliminate than other bacterial infections. If identified and treated in the first two stages (the most infectious stages), antibiotics are very effective.

   Stage 1 (primary)—characterized by circular sores called chancres. The center of these sores hold a pool of the virus, which is very infectious. After 5 to 6 weeks, the sores clear up and go away (with or without treatment).

   Stage 2 (secondary)—characterized by a rash that first shows up on the palms of the hands and the soles of the feet. Also, noticeable hair loss. Again, the rash will go away in about 5 weeks, with or without treatment.

Stage 3 (latent)—can last 20 to 30 years as the bacteria go dormant, BUT certain life circumstances can cause the bacteria to progress to the next stage.

Stage 4 (tertiary stage)—Now the spirochetes have spread around the body and have chosen an organ or area (eyes, brain, ears, heart, etc.) to infect. Without recognition and treatment, this can be fatal.

7. Trichomoniasis—Trichomonas vaginalis is a parasite that causes inflammation in the pelvic region, along with painful urination, itching, and discharge. Treated with topical medications and antibiotics.

8. Pubic lice—Parasites that live on the skin of other living creatures and feed on their blood. These are treated with topical medications. The pubic louse is smaller than head or body lice.

9. Scabies—Parasite that burrows under the skin, laying its eggs at the base of hair follicles. Treated with topical medications.

10. Hepatitis A, B, and C—A contagious disease that attacks the liver. Most cases are caused by a virus, but a few are caused by alcohol abuse, toxins, and some medications. Hepatitis A and B have vaccines, while Hepatitis C does not.

Hepatitis A—acute and rarely chronic. Occurs when one ingests food or water infected by someone else's stool. Mostly related to hygiene.

Hepatitis B—disproportionately affects Asian Americans and Pacific Islanders (AAPI). Occurs through contact with infected blood or blood products.

Hepatitis C—the most common route of infection comes from sharing needles. Symptoms are not very recognizable, so many go untreated. Over time the virus attacks the liver, causing liver damage later in life.

Pelvic inflammatory disease (PID)—The result of a number of untreated bacterial STIs. Symptoms include inflammation of organs of the reproductive system. This infection can result in sterility.

Reference

Kaufman, J. (2020). Sexually Transmitted Infections. Retrieved from https://my.wlu.edu/student-life/health-and-safety/student-health-and-counseling/health-library/stis

CHAPTER 16

NONCOMMUNICABLE DISEASE

Cardiovascular Disease (CVD)

The number one killer of adults in the United States is cardiovascular disease. There are multiple conditions categorized under CVD. To have a basic understanding of these conditions, one must have a basic understanding of the cardiovascular system.

Heart Anatomy

The heart has four chambers, two atria and two ventricles. The atria collect blood as it is pumped throughout the body, and the ventricles pump the blood out of the heart. The movement of blood throughout the body is cyclical and nonstop.

Beginning on the right side, deoxygenated blood flows into the **right atrium** via the **superior and inferior venae cavae.** It passes through the **tricuspid valve** into the **right ventricle**. The right ventricle pumps the deoxygenated blood out of the heart through the **pulmonary valve** to the **pulmonary arteries** and to the **lungs**, where it is oxygenated and pumped back to the heart via the **pulmonary veins**. The oxygen-rich blood enters the **left atrium** and goes through the **bicuspid valve (mitral valve)** into the **left ventricle**, through the **aortic valve** to the **aorta**, where it is pumped to the rest of the body.

The heart muscle, the **myocardium**, is responsible for pumping blood 24/7.

The body's pacemaker is a small bundle of cells that signal the heart to beat. It is located in the upper quadrant of the right atrium.

The left ventricle is the most muscular chamber of the heart due to its responsibility of pumping oxygenated blood out of the heart to the rest of the body.

Several factors contribute to heart health and heart disease. Some are modifiable, and some are not.

<u>Nonmodifiable Factors That Contribute to Heart Disease:</u>
Gender, age, ethnicity, genetics

<u>Modifiable Factors That Contribute to Heart Disease:</u>
High cholesterol and triglycerides, smoking, high blood pressure, obesity, lack of physical activity, diabetes, stress

Most Common Cardiovascular Diseases

The following is a list of the 12 most common cardiovascular diseases:

1. *Coronary artery disease (CAD)*—damage or narrowing of the coronary blood vessels responsible for supplying oxygenated blood to the myocardium.
2. *Arteriosclerosis*—degenerative changes in the blood vessels of the body.
3. *Atherosclerosis*—most common of the atherosclerotic conditions, where the blood vessels are clogged by fatty buildup and plaque.
4. *High blood pressure (HBP)*—changes in blood flow that require the heart to work harder in order to pump blood throughout the body. One of the easiest ways to chart heart health is to have your blood pressure taken. A reading of 120/80 is considered healthy.
5. *Cardiac arrest (myocardial infarction)*—sudden stoppage of the heartbeat.
    - *Cardiopulmonary resuscitation (CPR)*—Artificial pumping of the stopped heart, keeping the blood flow moving throughout the body, especially to the brain. Learning to perform CPR is a lifesaving skill.
6. *Congestive heart failure*—chronic condition where the heart doesn't move blood adequately, causing a fluid buildup in the lungs.
7. *Arrhythmia*—an irregular beating of the heart. Indicates a problem with the body's pacemaker.
    - Tachycardia—heartbeat is too fast
    - Bradycardia—heartbeat is too slow
8. *Peripheral vascular disease/peripheral artery disease (PVD/PAD)*—narrowed vessels in the body restrict blood flow to the arms and legs, causing stabbing pains and potential tissue death.
9. *Congenital heart defects*—anatomical defects in the heart that occur during fetal development. Present at birth.
10. *Cardiomyopathy*—heart muscle becomes inflamed and enlarged, making it too big for the chest cavity. This enlargement interferes with healthy heart function.
11. *Pericardial disease*—inflammation of the pericardium of the heart. The pericardium is a thin multilayer sac that protects the heart from infection.
12. *Heart valve disease*—valves maintain one-way blood flow through the heart. When there is a malformation or malfunction of these valves, you have the potential for life-threatening problems. Commonly referred to as a heart murmur.

Diagnosing and Treating CVDs:

- *Electrocardiogram (ECG)*—attaching electrodes to the chest to get a printout of the heart's electrical rhythm.

- *Echocardiogram*—determines the thickness of the heart muscle and how efficiently it is pumping.

- *Angiography*—dye is injected into a blood vessel in order to view its paths through the coronary arteries, looking for blockage or narrowing.

Treatments:

Angioplasty—inserting a small balloon into the partially blocked vessels and inflating it in order to open the narrowed passageway

Coronary bypass surgery—surgically bypassing the damaged artery with replacement vessels

Cardioversion—done for arterial fibrillation, using drug therapy or electrical shock. Both regulate the heartbeat.

Stroke

Sudden disruption of blood flow to the brain causing disability and possibly death.

Ischemic Stroke: An ischemia is the narrowing of a blood vessel. With this type of stroke, a partially blocked blood vessel becomes completely blocked by an embolism (traveling blood clot) or develops a complete closure.

Hemorrhagic Stroke: Rupture or blockage of blood vessels that supply the brain with oxygen and other nutrients. Within minutes, brain tissue will begin to die.

Transient Ischemic Attack (TIA): Sometimes called a mini-stroke. Temporary disruption of blood flow to the brain that does not cause permanent brain damage.

Diagnosing and Treating a Stroke

FAST

F—face droop

A—arm weakness or numbness

S—speech difficulty

T—time to call 911

Immediate treatment of a stroke can lessen the long-term effects. The IV administration of the clot-busting drug Activase (tPA) is one such treatment.

Diagnosing potential risks for stroke:

- Computerized tomography scan (CT scan)
- Magnetic resonance imaging (MRI)
- Electroencephalogram (EEG)

Stroke survivors may experience the following temporary or permanent disabilities:

- Paralysis or loss of muscle movement, dependent upon location of clot in the brain; usually happens to one side of the body or just the face

- Trouble speaking or swallowing

- Memory loss or thinking difficulties

- Emotional problems and/or behavioral changes; mood swings and depression

- Unexplainable pain and numbness

Stroke prevention strategies are similar to those that help prevent cardiovascular disease.

Cancer

The second-leading cause of adult deaths in the United States.

Cancer: Cells that mutate and divide, becoming abnormal. These cells attack healthy cells and can spread throughout the body via the blood stream and lymph system. The damaged cells bond together, forming growths or tumors.

There are over 100 types of cancers. The two most common causes for the development of these growths are genetics and exposure to carcinogens (cancer-causing agents).

Genetics: Cancer can run in families. If cancer is in your family tree, you should check if the cancer can be traced back to a modifiable lifestyle factor (see list under CVDs). If not, you may be predisposed to develop that type of cancer.

Carcinogens: Cancer-causing agents that we are exposed to in our environment and diet. These promote cancer development and growth.

The most common carcinogens are radiation (sun), smoking, poor diet, and some viruses or other infections. While studies have not shown obesity to cause cancer, there is consistent evidence that higher amounts of body fat are associated with increased risk of the following cancers: endometrial, esophageal, liver, kidney, multiple myeloma, brain, pancreatic, colorectal, gallbladder, ovarian, and thyroid (Musen, 2017).

Two Types of Cancerous Growths

Benign Tumors: Noncancerous; these tumors only become dangerous when they interfere with healthy cell function. Benign tumors include cysts, moles, warts, and other nonmalignant masses.

Malignant Tumors: Cancerous growths that interfere with healthy cell function. They can metastasize (invade other parts of the body).

Cancer Diagnosis

Self-Checks: Early detection depends on self-checks that can be done by the patient to help find unusual lumps. Especially effective in diagnosing breast cancer, skin cancer, and testicular cancer.

Biopsy: Removing a small piece of tissue from the tumor and sending it to a lab for evaluation. This can help determine the following classification:

TNM

T—the extent of the primary tumor (size)

N—the presence or absence of lymph node involvement

M—presence of metastasis

Stages I–IV: Stage I is the least invasive stage, while Stage IV can be terminal.

Cancer Treatment

Surgery: Invasive procedure where the doctor goes into the site of invasion and removes as much of the mass as possible.

Chemotherapy: Drug treatment via IV or oral pills for some cancers. Also used as a backup after surgery to make sure all of the mutated cells are gone. These drugs also damage healthy tissues.

Radiation: Used with chemotherapy and surgery as another backup to make sure all of the cancer is gone. A strong dosage of radiation is aimed at the site of the tumor for approximately 5 minutes. This type of treatment also damages healthy tissue.

Immunotherapy: Drug therapy used to stimulate the immune system to work harder and smarter to attack cancer cells. They add manmade immune system helpers such as specific proteins to destroy the mutant cells.

Self-Check: Manipulation of areas of the body, looking for unusual lumps or growths. Everyone should engage in this practice, especially focusing on the breasts and surrounding tissues and the testicles.

Chronic Diseases

Chronic disease is an umbrella term that incudes diseases that last longer than 1 year and that require ongoing medical attention and/or limit activities of daily living.

The NCBI (National Center for Biotechnology Information) warns that the definition for chronic disease varies within the medical community. The CDC, WHO, and Harvard Medical School all leave various diseases off the list for numerous reasons. This can become confusing for doctors when diagnosing a chronic condition (Raghupathi & Raghupathi, 2018).

The following diseases are the most common and show up on most of these lists:

Diabetes Mellitus: A disease of the pancreas. This condition affects how the body uses glycogen, our primary source of energy. This is the seventh leading cause of death in the United States.

<u>Prediabetes</u>—a blood test can determine if your sugar is too high, putting you at risk for diabetes.

<u>Type 1</u>—has been called "childhood" diabetes due to its early diagnosis. This type causes the pancreas to secrete too little insulin. Most people who suffer from this form of diabetes must inject insulin daily.

<u>Type 2</u>—is often called "adult onset" diabetes as it is usually diagnosed later in life and most times involves poor diet and issues with obesity. Unfortunately, today children as young as 12 are being diagnosed with this type of diabetes, mostly due to their weight. The pancreas does not process sugar efficiently, and the body has trouble keeping up with too much sugar/not enough insulin or too little sugar/too much insulin.

Symptoms—excessive thirst, increased urination, fatigue, blurred vision, slow-healing sores with frequent infections, weight loss with constant hunger, tingling in feet and hands, and red, tender gums.

Hyperglycemia—too much sugar/not enough insulin. Symptoms include headaches, dry mouth, fatigue, nausea, and fruity breath.

Hypoglycemia—not enough sugar/too much insulin. Symptoms include anxiety, pale skin, the shakes, sweating, hunger, and irritability.

If these symptoms continue for 2 weeks or longer, you need to see your doctor. Untreated diabetes can be life threatening.

Gestational Diabetes: Diagnosis of diabetes during pregnancy

Asthma: Mucus buildup in the bronchial passages of the lungs. This causes the airways to narrow, making it difficult to breathe. Symptoms are treated with inhalers.

Osteoarthritis: Joint pain or joint disease where the cushioning protecting the bone within the joint capsule dissolves. This disease is the leading cause of disability in the United States. The connection is clear: the more you weigh, the greater your risk is of developing this disease. Symptoms include swelling in the joints, pain, stiffness, and a decrease in range of motion. Treated with anti-inflammatory drugs and pain medications with eventual joint replacement.

Chronic Obstructive Pulmonary Disease (COPD): Blockage in the lungs, making breathing and the exchange of oxygen and carbon dioxide difficult. Smoking is the primary cause of COPD. This is the fourth leading cause of death in the United States.

Chronic bronchitis—regular buildup of mucus, making it difficult to get air into the lungs

Emphysema—destruction of alveoli, the primary conductors of gas exchange in the lungs

Inflammatory Bowel Disease (IBD): Disorders of the digestive tract

Crohn's disease—affects the lining of the digestive system, causing severe cramping, diarrhea, bloody stool, and lethargy. There is no cure for this disease, but treatment includes managing the diet by increasing fresh vegetables and fruits and eliminating nuts or beans, caffeine, and alcohol.

Ulcerative colitis—found mostly in the large intestine, this causes inflammation and ulcerations on the inner lining. Treated with anti-inflammatory and pain medications. Diet is very important to those living with this condition.

Parkinson's Disease: A neurodegenerative disease of the brain stem where the brain does not produce enough of the neurotransmitter dopamine. There is no cure, but treatment can improve quality of life. Parkinson's is terminal.

The most common symptom is uncontrollable shaking (tremors), along with limb rigidity, slowness of movement (bradykinesia), and gait and balance problems. Nonmotor symptoms include apathy, constipation, loss of smell, insomnia, depression, cognitive impairment, and hallucinations.

Lou Gehrig's Disease (Amyotrophic Lateral Sclerosis, or ALS): A progressive degeneration of motor neurons. Primarily affects the brain, nerve cells, and spinal cord.

Two types:

Sporadic—most common

Familial—5% to 10% of all cases in the United States; onset is at age 40

Multiple Sclerosis (MS): A disease of the central nervous system that disrupts the flow of information within the brain and between the brain and the body. Usually diagnosed between the ages of 20 to 50, with women 3 times more likely than men to be diagnosed.

Alzheimer's Disease: The most common type of dementia, it causes problems with memory, thinking, and behavior. Onset most commonly occurs after age 65. This is the sixth-leading cause of death in the United States.

Dementia is a general term for a decline in mental ability severe enough to interfere with daily functioning.

Alzheimer's is a progressive disease with no cure. In the early stages, symptoms include memory loss, especially newly learned information. As it advances through the brain, symptoms become more severe and include disorientation, mood and behavior changes, confusion, suspicious and paranoid behavior, and aggression.

Kidney Disease: Nephritis, nephrotic syndrome, and nephrosis. Affects 6 million adults in the United States, killing over 50,000 people a year.

Kidneys are one of the natural filters in the human body. Without them we cannot survive.

Treatments for kidney disease include dialysis or kidney transplant.

You are more likely to develop kidney disease if you have diabetes, high blood pressure, heart disease, or a genetic predisposition to kidney problems.

References

Musen, M. (2017). We Face a New "Tragedy of the Commons." The Remedy is Better Metadata. Comprehensive Cancer Information, National Cancer Institute. Retrieved on April 30, 2021, from https://www.cancer.gov/

Raghupathi, W., & Raghupathi, V. (2018). Chronic Disease Warning. An Empirical Study of Chronic Diseases in the United States: A Visual Analytics Approach to Public Health. International and Public Health. https://www.ncbi.nlm.nih.gov/pmc/articles/PMC5876976/

SOCIAL VIOLENCE

CHAPTER 17

RELATIONSHIP VIOLENCE

V IOLENCE IS A SERIOUS PROBLEM IN the United States. It affects every aspect of the society in which we live. In 1979, the US surgeon general identified violent behavior as a key public health priority.

In 1992, the Centers for Disease Control and Prevention (CDC) established the National Center for Injury Prevention and Control (NCIPC). Its primary focus is violence prevention.

National Domestic Violence Hotline: 1-800-799-7233.

Most commonly known as domestic violence (DV), intimate partner violence (IPV) involves violent behavior between two people who are in an intimate relationship. This pattern of behavior is used to gain or maintain power and control over an intimate partner.

Violent and abusive behavior is included as a public health priority area by the CDC in the Healthy People Studies conducted at the start of each decade since 1980.

In the United States, more than 10 million adults experience domestic violence or stalking by an intimate partner during their lifetime. That's 1 every 3 seconds. As many as 1 in 4 women and 1 in 10 men are victims of this type of violence.

From 2016 to 2018, the number of intimate partner violence (IPV) victimizations in the United States increased by 42%. On a typical day, domestic violence hotlines nationwide receive over 19,000 calls (Coalition Against Domestic Violence, 2020).

In an attempt to better understand relationship violence, the Domestic Abuse Intervention Project in Duluth, Minnesota, developed the Power and Control Wheel. This wheel is divided into nine pieces describing the many facets of relationship abuse. They are as follows:

1. Emotional abuse
2. Economic abuse
3. Using social status/privilege
4. Using children
5. Physical abuse
6. Denying, minimizing, and blaming
7. Intimidation and threats
8. Isolation and extreme jealousy
9. Sexual abuse

Recognizing that you or someone you care for is in this type of relationship is not easy, but there are warning signs that should alert you to this problem. Warning signs include the following:

1. Your partner humiliates you or puts you down.
2. Your partner makes you feel bad about yourself.
3. Your partner controls what you do, who you see, and where and how you spend money.
4. Your partner prevents you from getting or keeping a job.
5. Your partner tells you it's your fault when they hurt you.
6. Your partner uses your children to make you feel guilty or threatens to hurt the children.
7. Your partner threatens to take the children away from you.

If you recognize one or more of these signs but are afraid to discuss them with your partner, you must seek help. These behaviors will only escalate as time goes on.

According to the National Domestic Violence Hotline (2020), ways to offer your support to someone who is experiencing this type of abuse are as follows:

1. If there is denial, approach the topic gently.
2. If the person has confided in you, believe them.
3. Respect what they are going through and be nonjudgmental.
4. Reassure them that they are not alone and that you are there to support them.
5. Give them space to discuss it as little or as much as they need.
6. Acknowledge how difficult the situation is and emphasize that you are there to help.
7. Whatever outside resources or suggestions you offer, make clear you know the decision is theirs.
8. Help them come up with an SOS plan so that they can alert you in an emergency.
9. Offer to store clothes and personal items as safely as possible so that they can be retrieved in a hurry.
10. If they go in and out of the relationship, understand this is common and continue to support them.
11. Encourage them to seek support from loved ones and professionals.
12. Take care of yourself, and reach out for advice if you need it.
13. If you witness physical abuse directly, call 911. Never intervene in a violent altercation.

There are agencies in every major city in the United States that are funded solely to assist people in these situations.

Spousal Rape (Wife Abuse): In the 17th century, Sir Matthew Hale, an English jurist, theorized that a wife gave "irrevocable consent" to her husband. "By their mutual matrimonial consent and contract, the wife hath given up herself in this kind unto her husband which she cannot retract." It became illegal to beat your wife in 1920, and marital rape wasn't recognized as a crime in the United States until 1993. "More than 1 in 7 women who have ever been married have been raped" (National Clearinghouse on Marital and Date Rape, 2005).

References

Coalition Against Domestic Violence. (2020). https://assets.speakcdn.com/assets/2497/domestic_violence-2020080709/350855.pdf?1596811079991

National Clearinghouse on Marital and Date Rape. (2005, May). University of Pennsylvania, Department of Criminology. https://www.crim.sas.upenn.edu

National Domestic Violence Hotline. (2020). Ways to Support. A little help can go a long way. Retrieved on November 2, 2020, from: https://www.thehotline.org/support-others/ways-to-support/

CHAPTER 18

SOCIAL VIOLENCE

Hate Crimes

Hate Crimes (Bias-motivated Crime): Crimes motivated by the victim's actual or perceived race, ethnicity, national origin, sexual orientation, gender, religion, or disability. A criminal expression of bigotry.

The first bias-motivated crime statute in the United States was passed at the federal level by the Department of Justice in 1968. This law made the penalty more severe but was NOT labeled as "hate crime legislation."

The term *hate crime* was first used in the United States in the 1980s to describe a series of incidents aimed at Jews, Asians, and Blacks. In 1981, Washington and Oregon were the first states to pass hate crime legislation. Today, 49 states have hate crime statutes on their books. States vary on the groups included under these laws, along with the enhanced penalty handed down for committing a hate crime.

In 1998, the following two hate-motivated murders promoted the need for more legislation regarding hate crimes.

James Byrd Jr. (a Black man) was brutally murdered in Jasper, Texas, by three White supremacists. All three suspects were apprehended; two were sentenced to death, and one was given life in prison without the possibility of parole.

Matthew Shepard (a gay man) was brutally beaten and left to die, tied to a fence in Laramie, Wyoming. Since Wyoming did not have hate crime legislation when this crime was committed, the two suspects were sentenced to two life terms in prison.

In 2009, the Matthew Shepard and James Byrd Jr. Hate Crimes Prevention Act was passed. This was the first federal law to identify *hate crimes* as a more severe type of assault. It was improved upon by the Obama administration in 2010.

The FBI defines a hate crime as "a criminal offense committed against a person, property, or society that is motivated, in whole or in part, by the offender's bias against a race, religion, disability, sexual orientation, or ethnicity/national origin."

Prevalence of hate crimes: In 2019, 57.6% of reported hate crimes were racially motivated; 20.1% were religiously motivated; and 16.7% were motivated by perceived sexual orientation (U.S. Department of Justice, 2019).

Enhanced penalties for hate crimes: For crimes using guns, explosives, fire, or other weapons, the offender can get up to 10 years in prison. Enhanced penalties for kidnapping, sexual assault, and murder can bring life in prison (no parole) or the death penalty.

Rape

Rape is sexual assault, not limited to forced intercourse. This crime is not gender specific, although more women than men are raped. This is an underreported crime due to the stigma it carries. Those who have been raped are often not believed and brutally questioned about the crime. If you have been raped, it is very important to go to a medical facility as soon as you are able. There they can perform a rape kit to collect evidence that will identify the offender. Without this evidence, it becomes the victim's word against the offender's.

Statutory Rape: Sexual contact with a person who is under the age of consent (a minor). This definition varies from state to state.

RAINN—Rape, Abuse, and Incest National Network

This is the nation's largest anti–sexual violence organization. It offers programs to prevent sexual violence, help survivors, and ensure that perpetrators are brought to justice.

Elder Abuse

Elder Abuse National Hotline: 1-800-510-2020

For seniors over age 65 in the United States, abuse and neglect are serious issues. Approximately 1 in 6 seniors are the victims of some type of abuse. Many cases go unreported, which makes this a difficult crime to track. Elder and dependent adult abuse is not uncommon in our society. Abuse can come in different forms, such as physical, emotional, financial, and neglect. Whether at home, living with family members, or in a care facility, these types of abuse are easily hidden.

A caregiver is any person who has assumed care or legal custody of a dependent adult, regardless of compensation. Many times, these caregivers are the dependent adult's children or other immediate family members. If abuse is occurring, the victim is hesitant to report it due to embarrassment or fear of retaliation.

Signs of abuse may include any or all of the following:

- Physical injuries
- Dramatic changes in the behavior of the victim
- Depression, unusual fear, or withdrawal
- Financial losses
- Missing items
- Hygiene issues (lack of bathing and washing hair, dirty clothes)

- Alcohol use
- Obvious weight loss
- Missing necessities (eyeglasses, walker, hearing aid, etc.) (National Institute on Aging, 2020)

Child Abuse

National Child Abuse Hotline: 1-800-422-4453 or www.childhelp.org

When a parent or legal guardian, through action or inaction, causes physical, sexual, and/or emotional harm to a child or the death of a child, this is child abuse. This also includes exploitation and neglect.

Every year more than 3 million reports of child abuse are made in the United States. Studies show that 1 in 4 girls and 1 in 8 boys are sexually abused before the age of 18.

While no child invites abuse, some are more at risk than others. These risk factors include the following:

- Mental or physical disabilities
- Social isolation of the family
- Parents lack understanding of raising children
- Parents have history of abuse
- Family is socioeconomically disadvantaged
- Family dysfunction
- Parental mental illness

Child abuse can be reported using hotlines available all over the country by anyone who suspects that a child is in danger.

If you are a mandated reporter, you are legally required to report reasonable suspicion of abuse of a child. Government employees, teachers, daycare workers, and law enforcement all fall into this category.

Some children may exhibit signs of child abuse, such as fear of complaining or talking to adults due to threats made by their abuser. They are also afraid that no one will believe their word over an adult's word.

Many times, it is necessary to seek medical attention to determine if some form of abuse is happening.

In 2018, David (age 56) and Louise (age 49) Turpin were arrested for one of the largest child abuse crimes of this decade. The Turpins lived in Perris, California, with their 13 children, ranging in age from 2 to 29. The parents were accused of torture, neglect, starvation, strangulation, physical abuse, sexual abuse, and false imprisonment. They both pled not guilty, but were eventually found guilty of these crimes and are now serving life in prison.

On a Sunday morning, their 17-year-old daughter was able to escape the family home with a deactivated cell phone and called 911. She alerted the police to the horrendous conditions that they were living in and were able to give them an address. When the sheriffs arrived, they were stunned and appalled by what they found.

Several of the children were chained (with padlocks) to their beds. All but the two-year-old appeared to be malnourished and were filthy. The house reeked of feces and urine, and there did not appear to be any food or water directly available to any of the children.

The neighbors reported rarely seeing the children, but when they did, the children did not look healthy, being very underweight and having pasty-white skin tone. The children reported that they were told to sleep all day and do housework and yardwork at night. They were fed on a strict schedule and were given the bare necessities for nutrition. David would buy apple pies and other treats and put them up where the children could see them, but they were never allowed to eat them. Those were saved for the parents.

Today the children (seven of whom are now adults) are recovering in foster homes in and around Southern California.

How can you tell if a child is being abused? Look for these behaviors or signs:

- Unexplained changes in behavior or personality
- Becoming withdrawn
- Seeming anxious
- Becoming uncharacteristically aggressive
- Lacks social skills and has few friends
- Poor bond relationship with a parent
- Knowledge of adult issues inappropriate for their age

Human Trafficking

To report suspicious activity, call: 1-866-347-2423
National Human Trafficking Hotline: 1-888-373-7888

Human trafficking is the use of force, fraud, or coercion to obtain some type of labor or commercial sex act.

Victims are lured into trafficking situations by the use of violence, manipulation, false promises of well-paying jobs or romantic relationships. A "Romeo" is someone who gets the victim to trust him or her with attention, gifts, and promises of a better life. Those most susceptible to being victimized may have psychological or emotional vulnerability, economic hardships, lack of a social safety net, or are experiencing political instability in their country of origin.

<u>Myths</u> concerning human trafficking:

- Human trafficking only happens in other countries
- Victims are either foreigners with poor English-language skills or are poor
- Human trafficking and human smuggling are the same thing
- Human trafficking victims will attempt to seek help when in public

All of the above are misconceptions and untrue regarding human trafficking.

Identifying victims: The following are some of the signs to look for when evaluating possible victims.

- Has the person disconnected from family and friends?

- Has the person had a sudden change in behavior?

- Does the person show signs of mental or physical abuse?

- Does the person seem fearful, timid, or submissive?

- Does the person keep company with someone who seems to be in control?

- Does the person lack personal possessions and appear to have unstable living conditions?

Mass Shootings (Gun Violence)

A mass shooting is defined as any incident in which four or more people are killed along with the shooter.

The gun homicide rate in the United States is 25 times higher than our peer countries. This difference has been attributed to our easy access to guns.

States within the United States with weaker gun laws and higher gun ownership rates have higher rates of mass shootings. One in three mass shooters are legally prohibited from possessing firearms at the time of the shooting. In 56% of mass shootings, the shooter exhibited dangerous warning signs before the shooting.

In the 10 years between 2009 and 2018, 1,121 were shot and killed in the United States in a mass shooting, and 836 more were shot and wounded. When assault weapons are used in a mass shooting, 6 times as many people are shot (EverytownUSA.org., 2019).

Examples of these shootings: These are just six examples of mass shootings that have occurred over the years. Seemingly, the event that kicked off this phenomenon were the shootings at Columbine High school in Colorado in April of 1999. The two shooters, students from the high school, entered the school and began shooting. They eventually killed 33 people, including themselves.

- The Harvest Music Festival shooting in Las Vegas, Nevada. In October of 2017, a 64-year-old man shot and killed 58 people from a hotel room overlooking the festival. He later killed himself.

- On June 17, 2015, a 26-year-old man went to a church in Charleston, South Carolina, where he prayed with parishioners for over an hour before opening fire and killing nine of them. He is serving life in prison.

- On December 15, 2012, a 20-year-old man entered Sandy Hook Elementary school in Newtown, Connecticut, and shot 26 people; 20 of them were six- and 7-year-old children. He then took his own life.

- On December 2, 2015, in San Bernardino, California, a man and a woman opened fire on employees at one of the shooters' workplace. They killed 14 people and wounded 24 before being killed in a shootout with police.

- In November of 2019, a 16-year-old gunman shot and killed four classmates outside of his high school in Santa Clarita, California. He later killed himself.

There have been too many of these shootings to list here, but the tide is not changing. These shootings continue all over the country, with efforts to stop them severely hampered by inadequate gun laws.

Across the country, gun laws vary by state. States with less restrictive policies regarding gun ownership, possession, and use show higher homicide rates. While the average number of deaths by shooting in the United States is 11.4 per 100,000 people, Alaska averages the most (22.2) and Massachusetts has the least (3.3).

According to Everytown.org research, these are some statistics regarding gun violence in the United States:

- Average deaths per year = 37,603

- The gun homicide rate in the United States is 25 times higher than that of other high-income countries.

- Gun homicides are concentrated in urban communities, and Black Americans represent the majority of victims.

- Access to a gun doubles the risk of homicide by gun.

- Approximately 3 million children witness gun violence every year.

- Every day, more than 100 Americans are shot and killed in the United States. (Everytown.org., 2019)

References

Everytown.org. (2019). Mass Shootings in the U.S. Retrieved from https://www.everytown.org/issues/mass-shootings/

National Institute on Aging (NIA). (2020, July 29). https://www.nia.nih.gov/health/elderabuse

U.S. Department of Justice. (2019). 2019 Hate Crime Statistics. Retrieved from https://ucr.fbi.gov/hate-crime/2019